MW00737332

My Baby's
1st Year

igloobooks

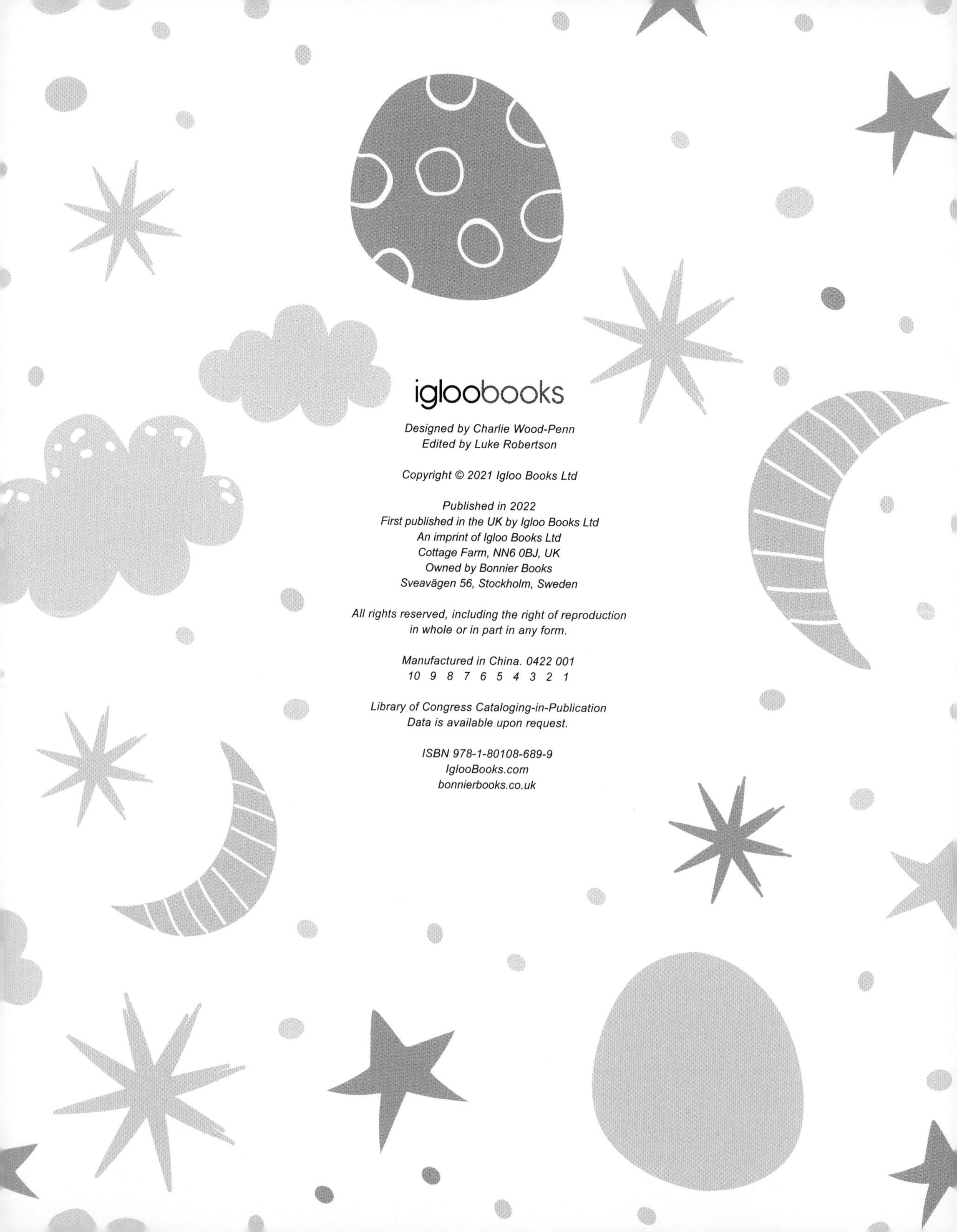

igloobooks

Designed by Charlie Wood-Penn
Edited by Luke Robertson

Published in 2022
First published in the UK by Igloo Books Ltd
An imprint of Igloo Books Ltd
Cottage Farm, NN6 0BJ, UK
Owned by Bonnier Books
Sveavägen 56, Stockholm, Sweden

Manufactured in China. 0422 001
10 9 8 7 6 5 4 3 2 1

Library of Congress Cataloging-in-Publication Data is available upon request.

ISBN 978-1-80108-689-9
IglooBooks.com
bonnierbooks.co.uk

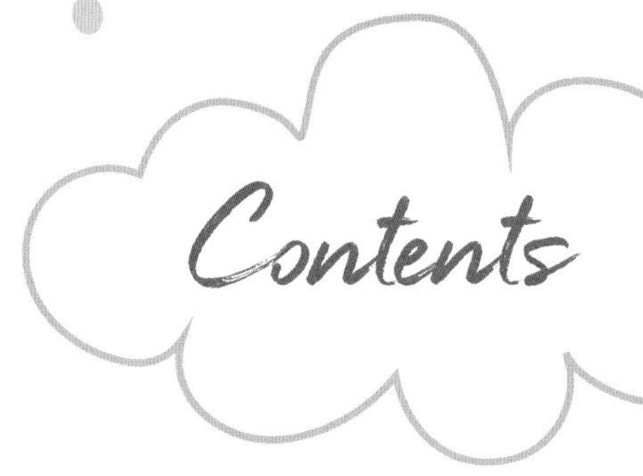

Contents

Before you were born 4
Important people you need to meet 16
Waiting for you to arrive 18
Hello, little one! 20
Look how small you were! 24
Coming home 26
Your fabulous firsts 30
1 month 36
2 months 39
3 months 42
4 months 45
5 months 48
6 months 51
7 months 55
8 months 58
9 months 61
10 months 65
11 months 68
12 months 71
Your first birthday! 77
Special occasions 84
Our trips 88
Our best pictures from this year 92

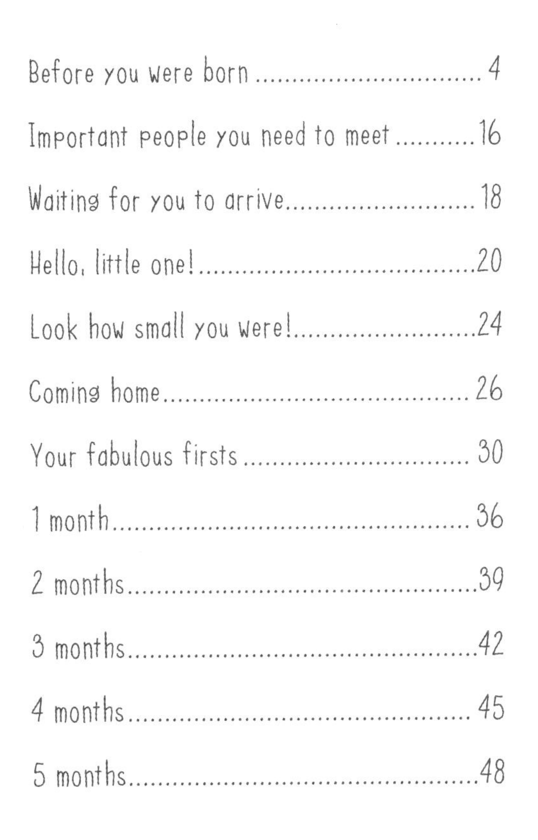

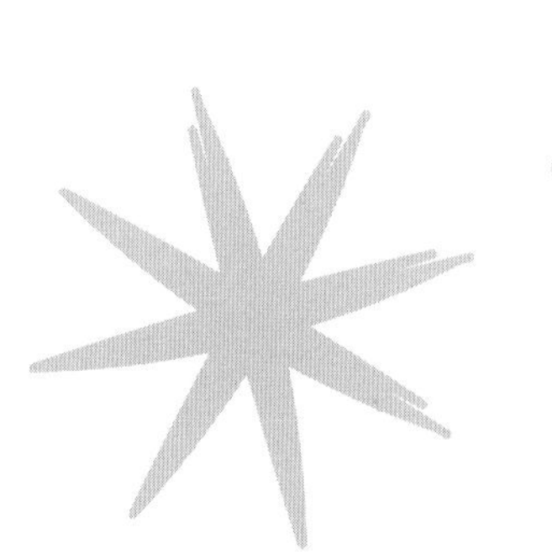

Before you were born

The day we found out you were coming

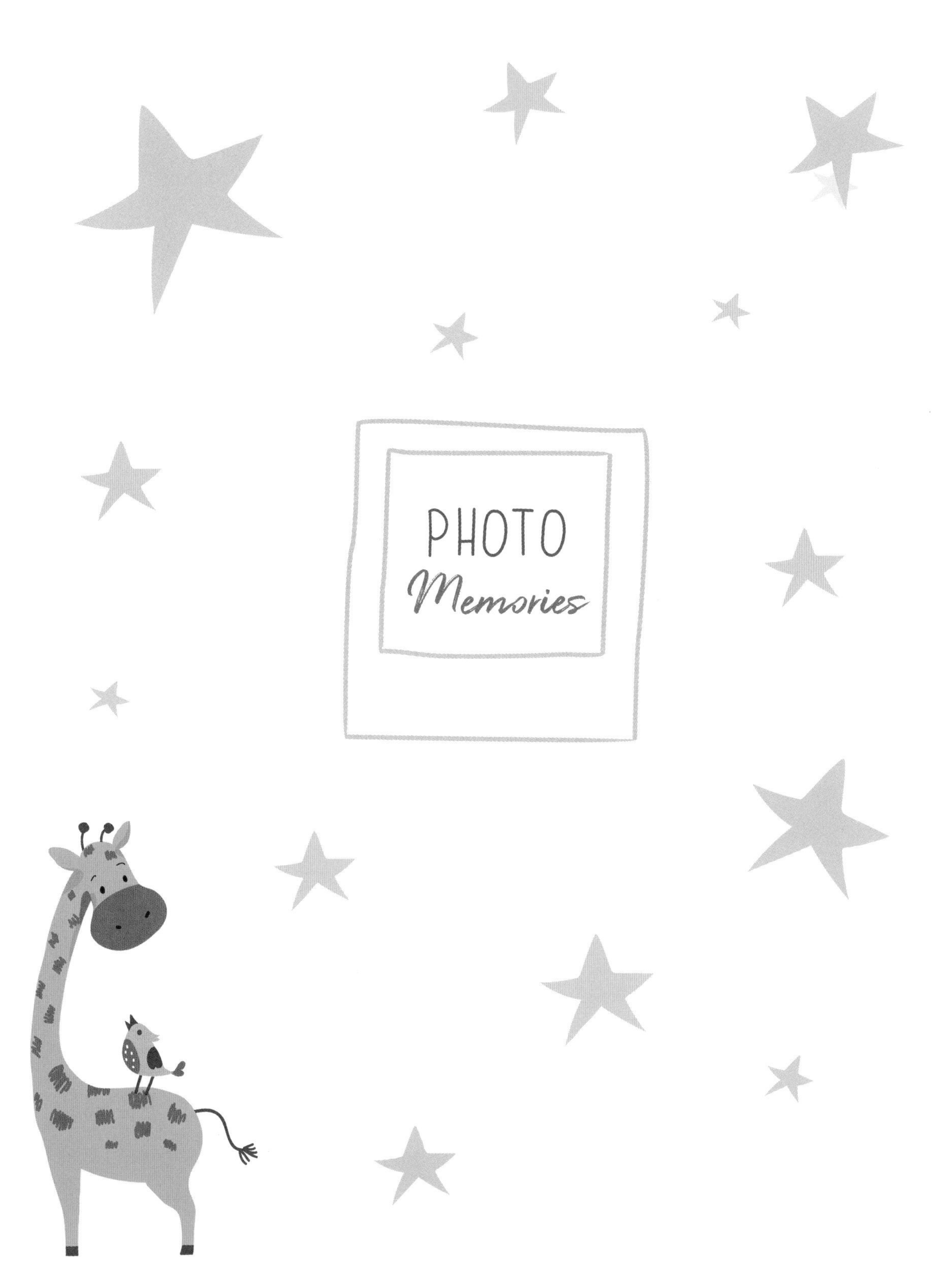
PHOTO
Memories

We are your parents

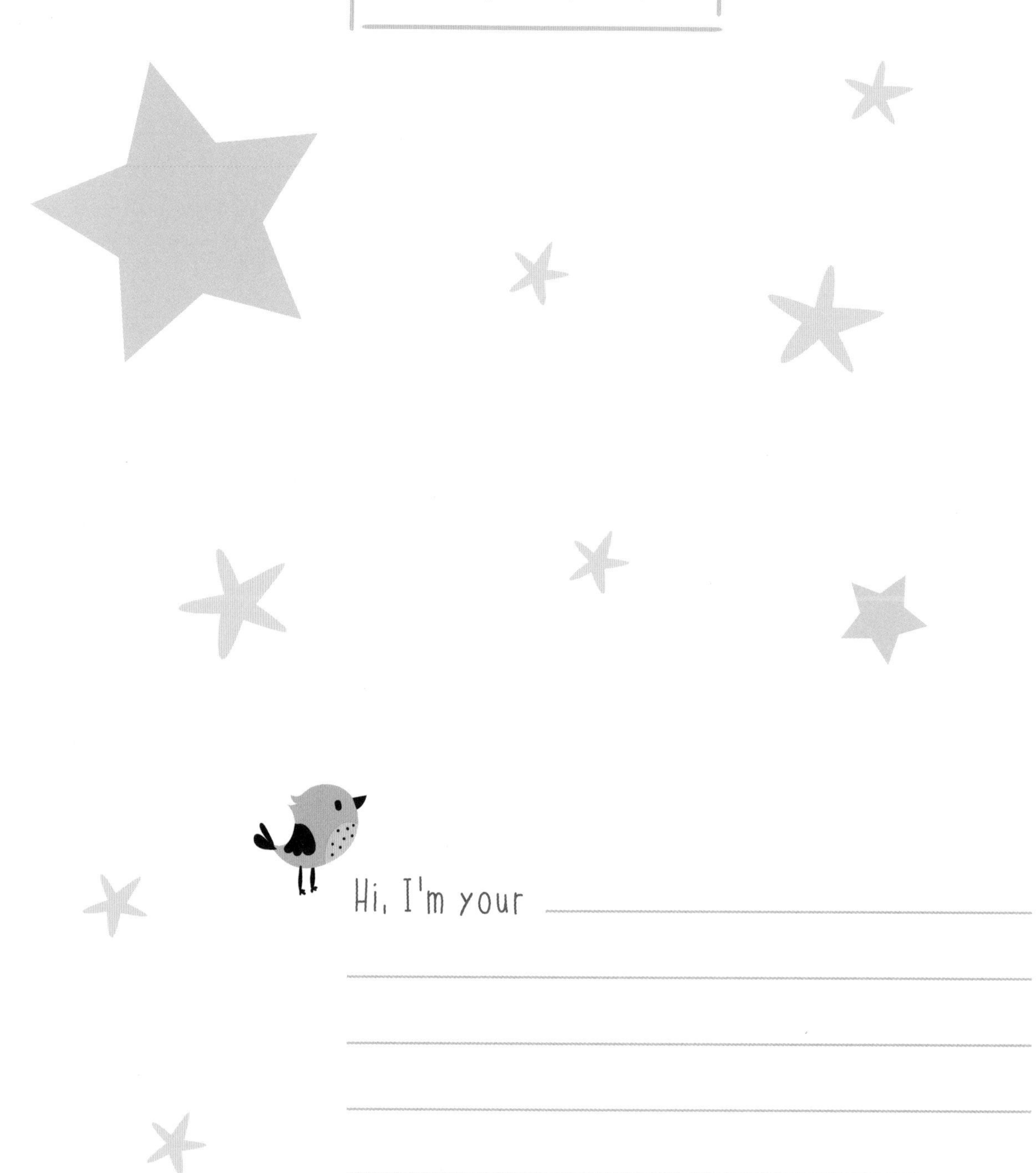

Hi, I'm your

Hi, I'm your

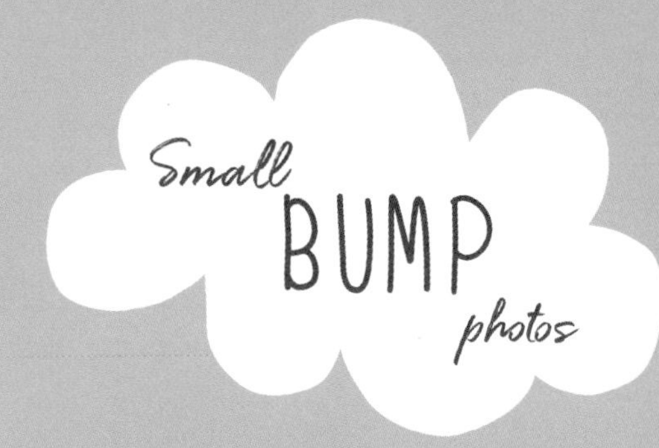
Small
BUMP
photos

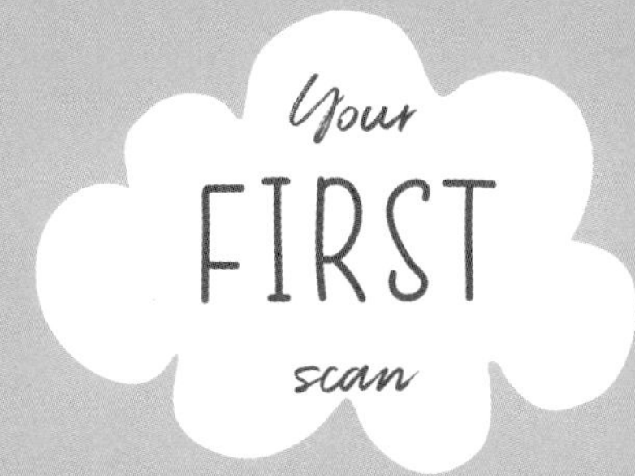
Your
FIRST
scan

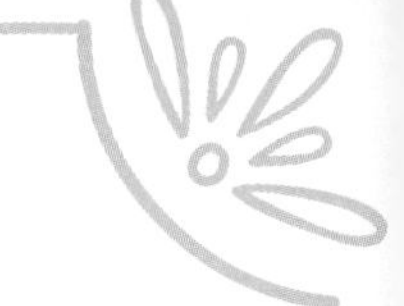
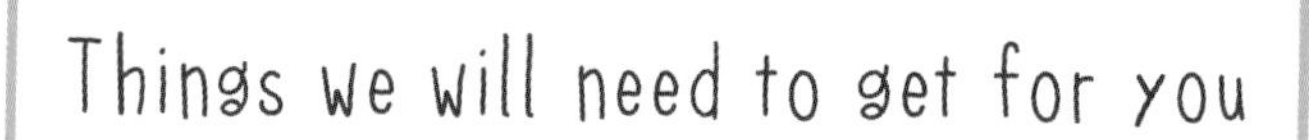

Things we will need to get for you

1.
2.
3.
4.
5.
6.
7.
8.
9.
10.
11.
12.
13.
14.
15.
16.
17.
18.
19.
20.

Getting ready for you to arrive

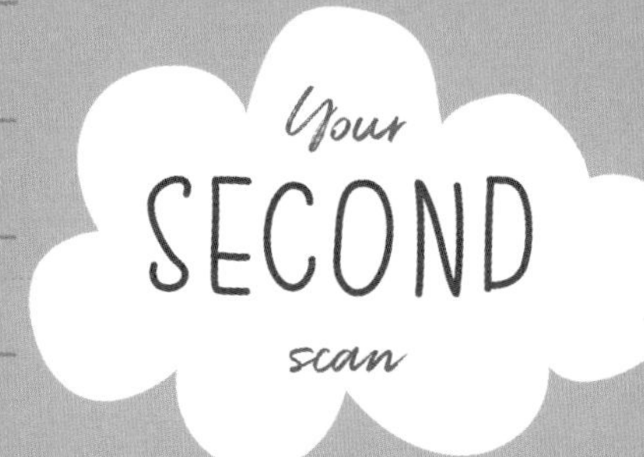
Your
SECOND
scan

Big BUMP Photos

BIGGER
bump photos

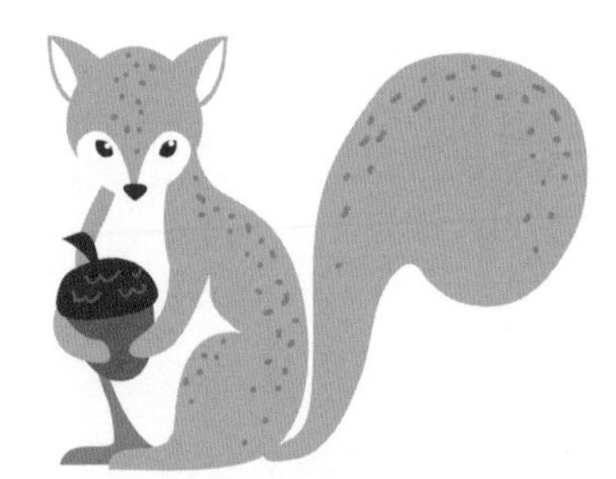

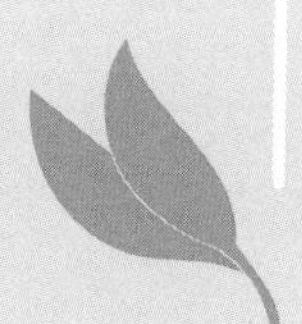

Name ideas

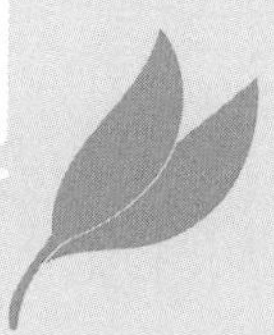

Important people you need to meet

Waiting for you to arrive

I hope that you

I hope you love

I hope you never forget

I hope you grow

I hope you become

I hope

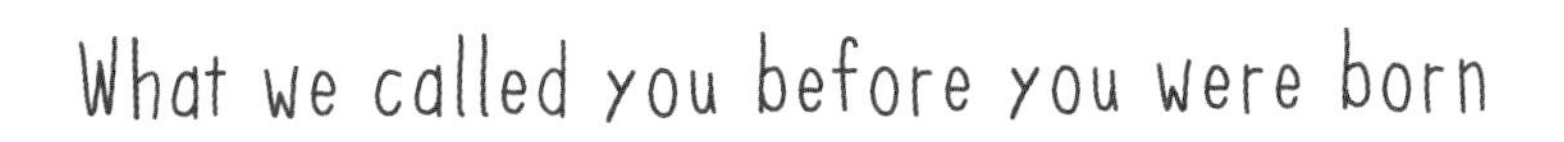

What we called you before you were born

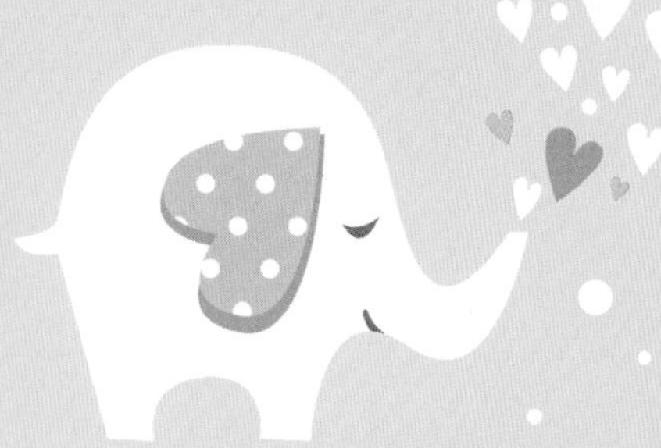

Hello, little one!

Date of birth ______________________

You were born . . . early [ ] on time [ ] late [ ]

Your eyes were ______________________

Your hair was ______________________

Our first moments with you ______________________

____

____

____

____

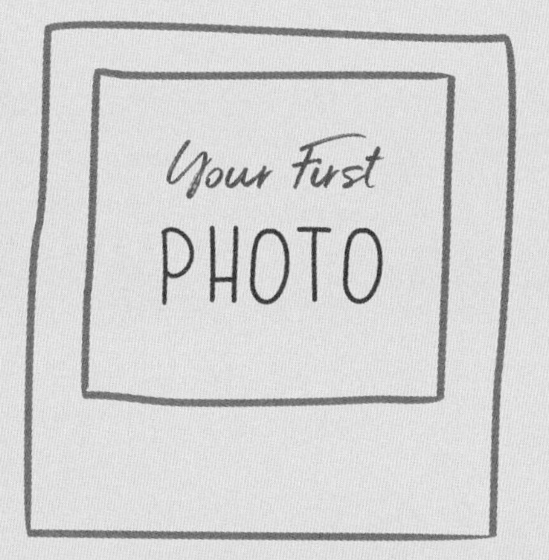
Your First
PHOTO

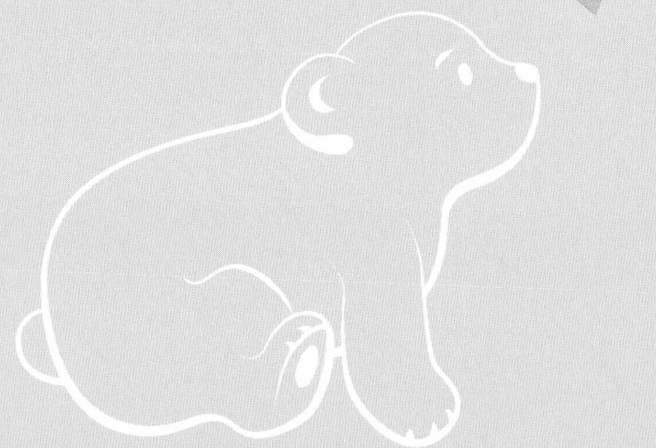

How we spent our first day together

Look how small you were!

Handprint

Date

You weighed

Your length was

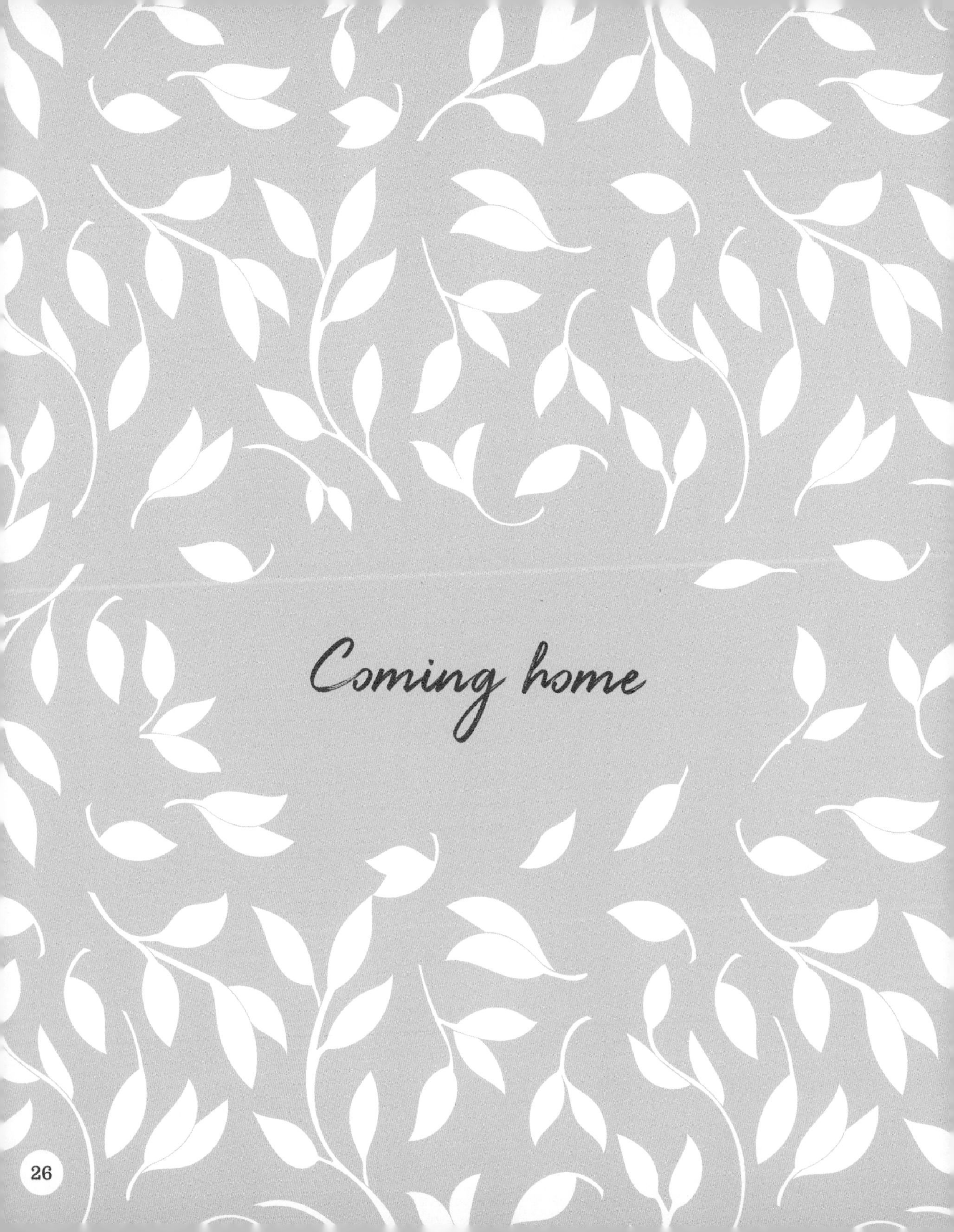

Coming home

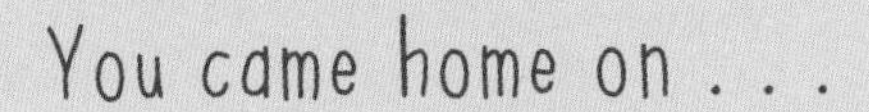

You came home on . . .

This was the photo we sent to tell people you were here!

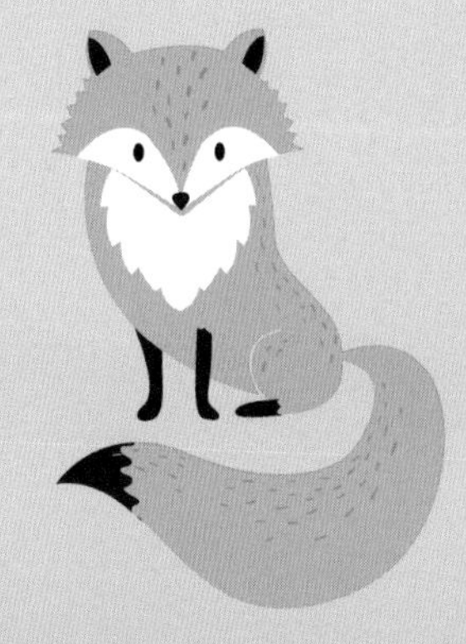

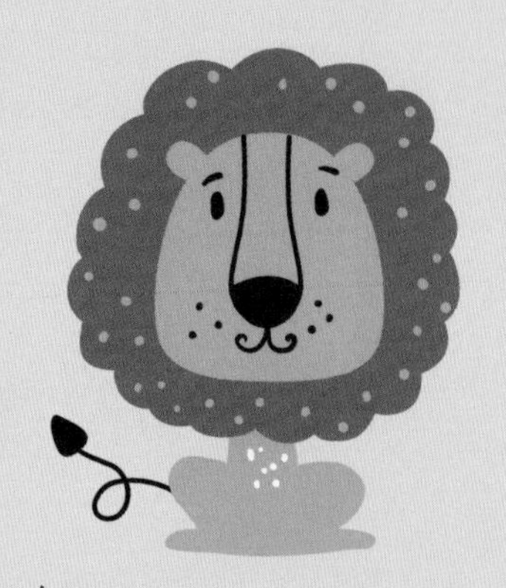

This is your nursery

This is your home

Your fabulous firsts

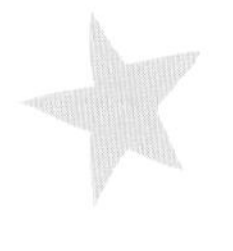

First visitors

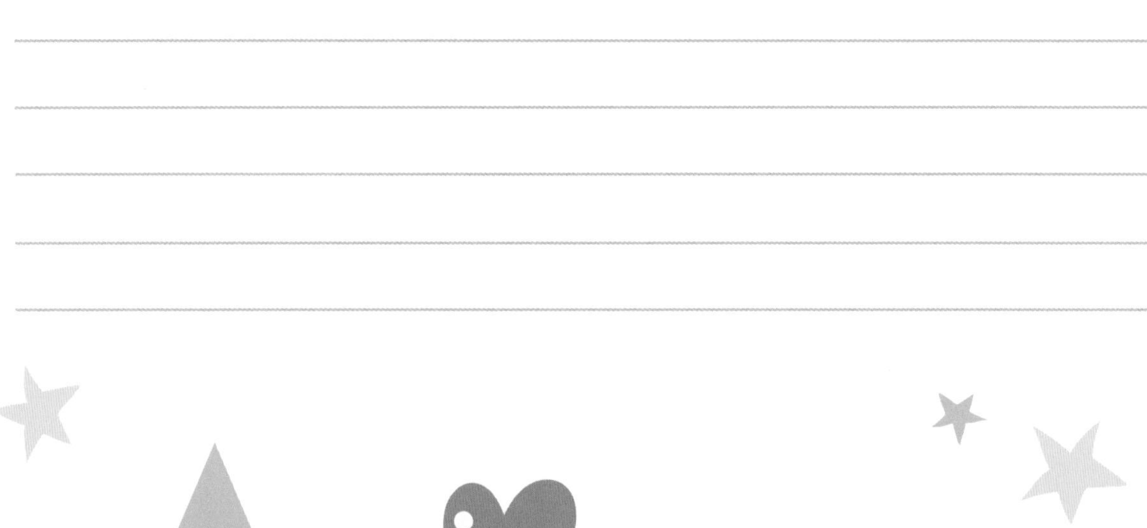

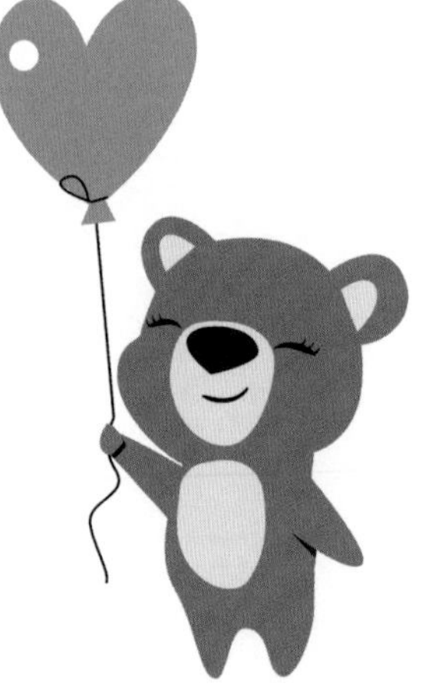

First bath

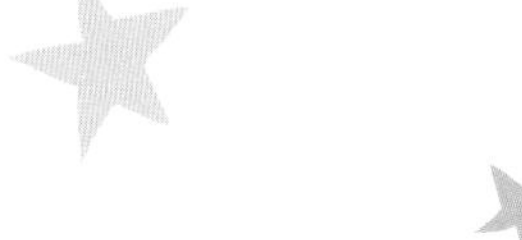

First time you sat up

First time you rolled over

First time you crawled

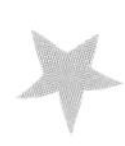

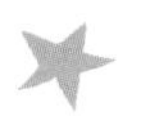

First time you stood up

First time you walked

First time you smiled

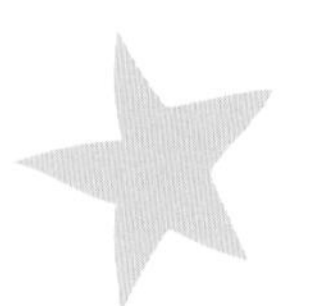

First time you laughed

Your first word

Your first solid food

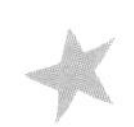

First time you clapped

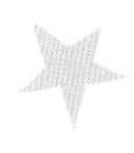

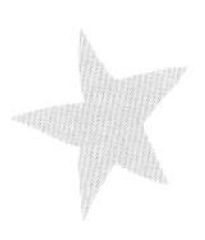

Your first tooth

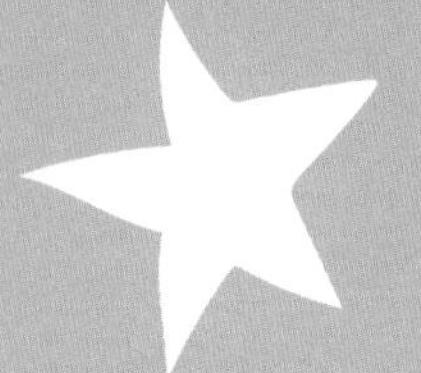

Your first haircut

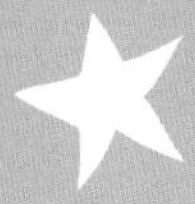

First time you slept in your own room

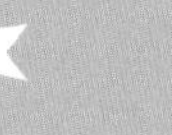

First time you slept through the night

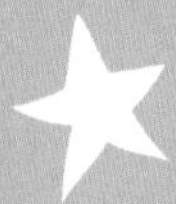

First time staying with someone else

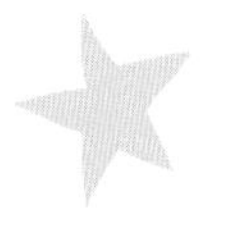

First day out

First holiday

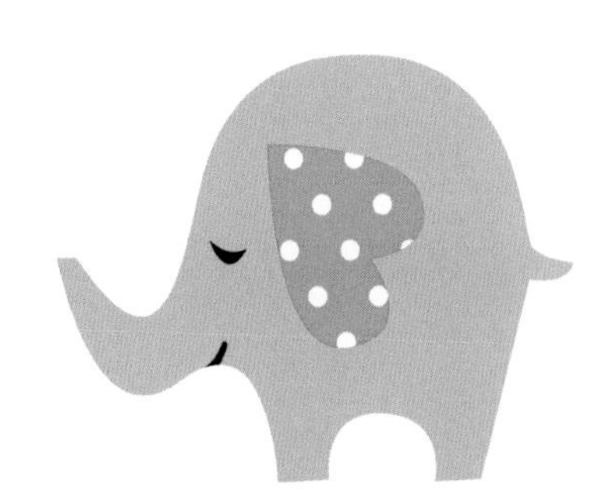

1 month

We did lots of . . .

This month you learned how to . . .

You're growing!

This is how much you grew!

2 months

PHOTO
Memories

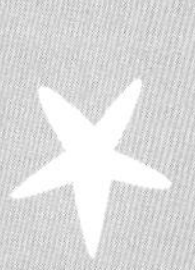

This month you learned how to . . . ______________________

____

____

____

____

____

We did lots of . . . ______________________

____

____

____

____

____

You're growing!

This is how much you grew!

3 months

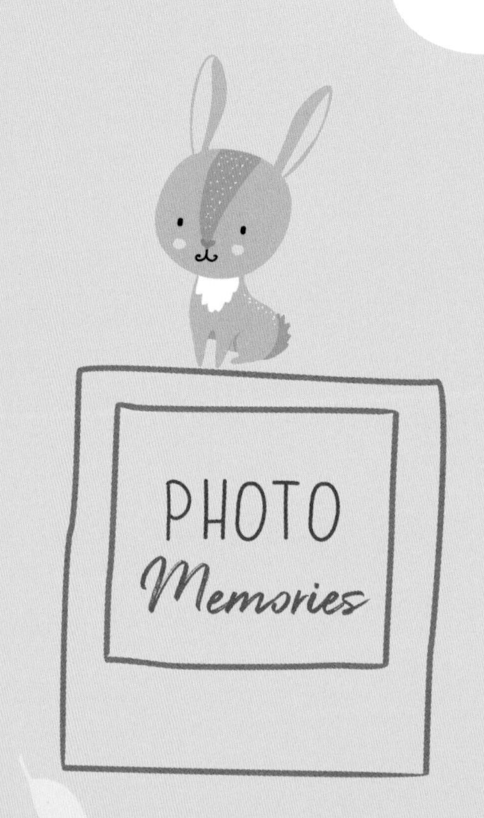

This month you learned how to . . .

We did lots of . . .

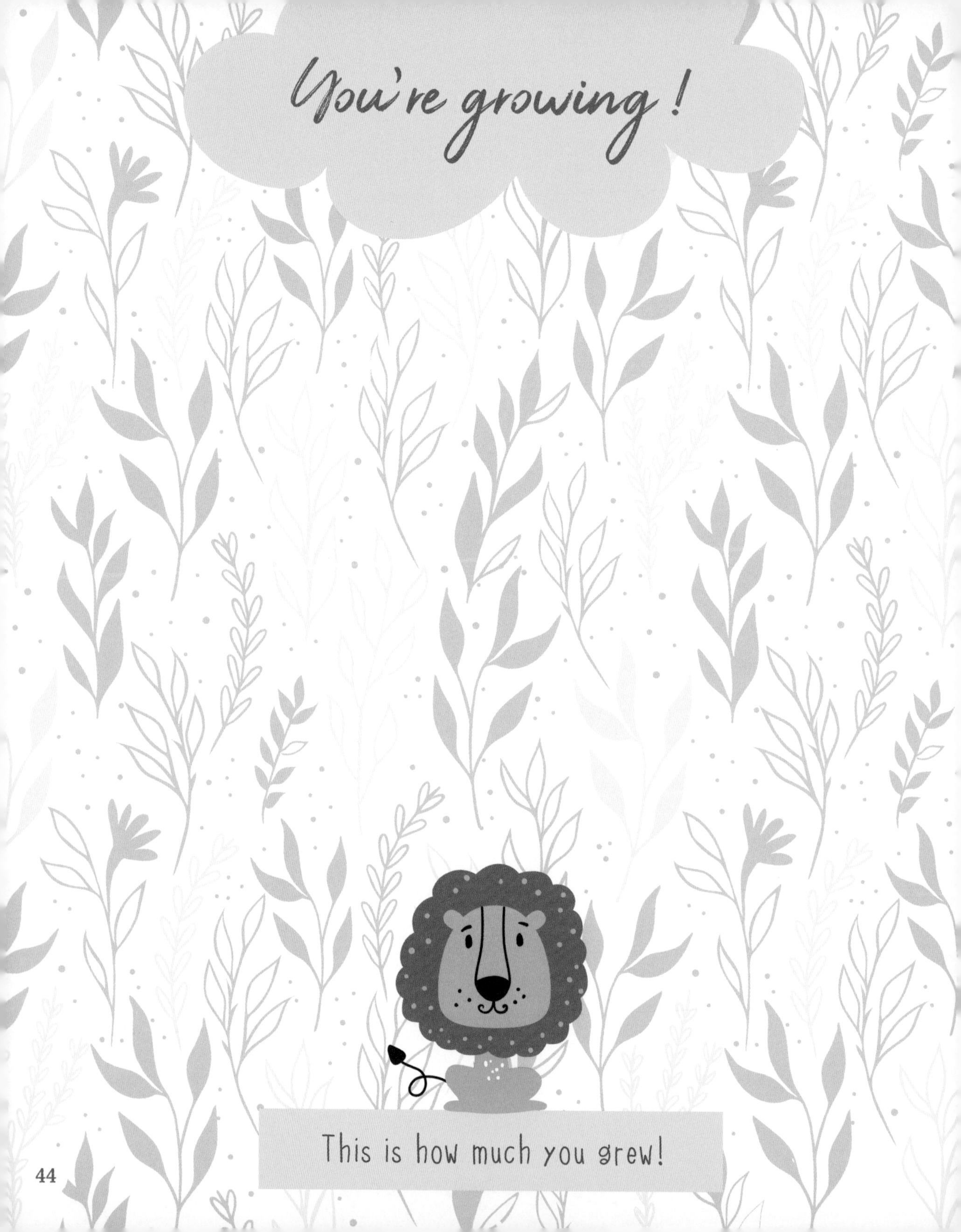
You're growing !
This is how much you grew!

4 months

This month you learned how to . . .

We did lots of . . .

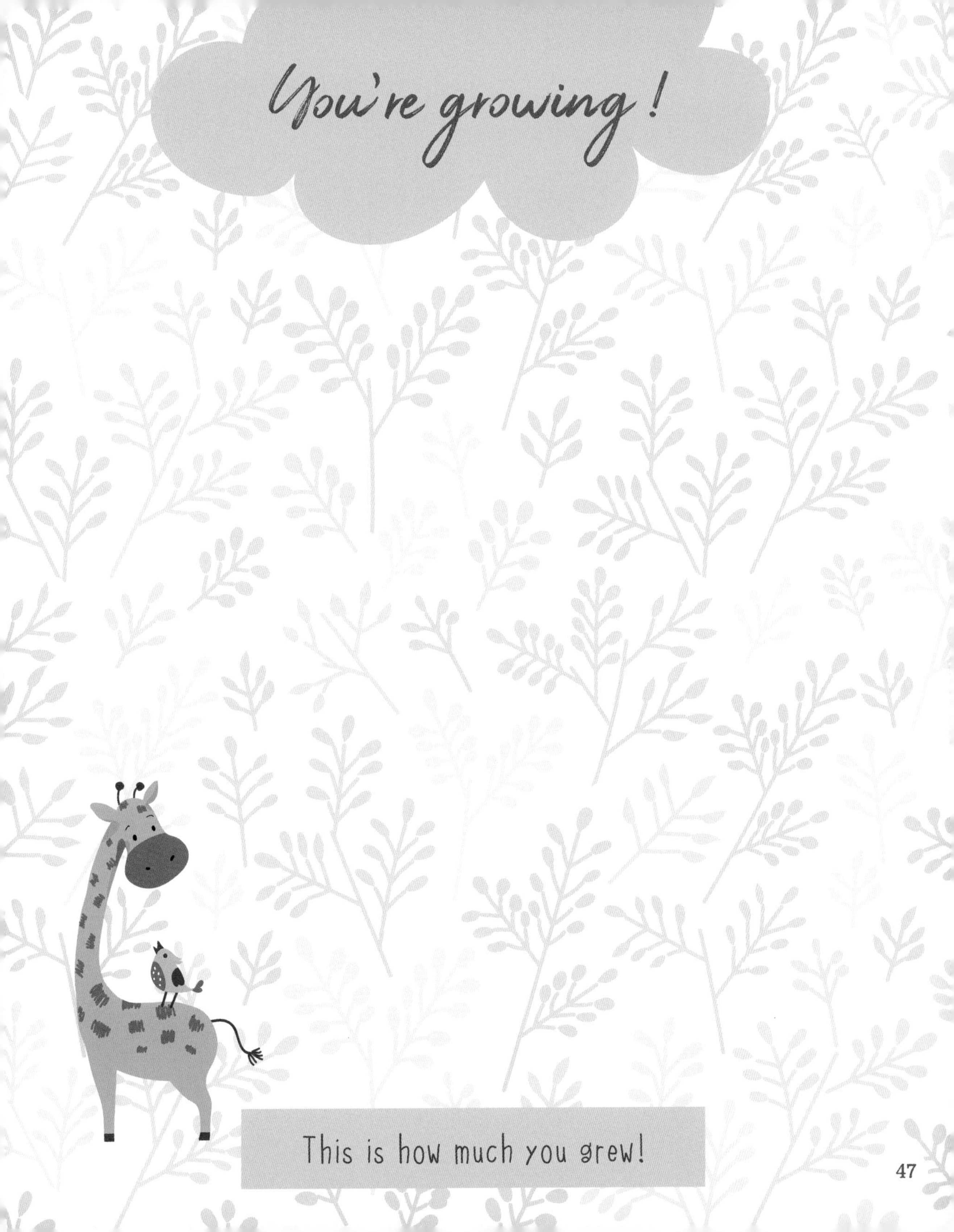
You're growing!
This is how much you grew!

5 months

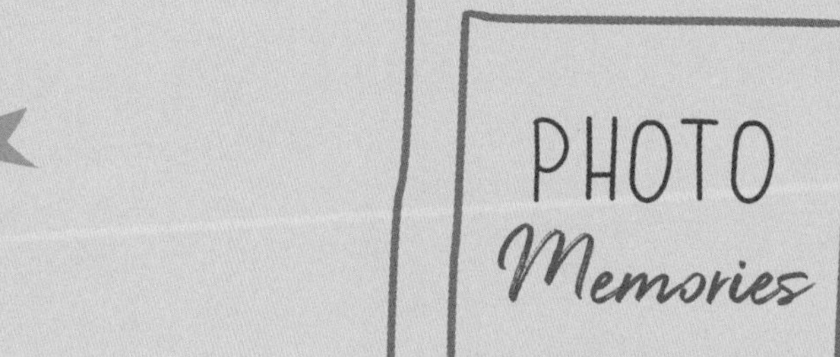

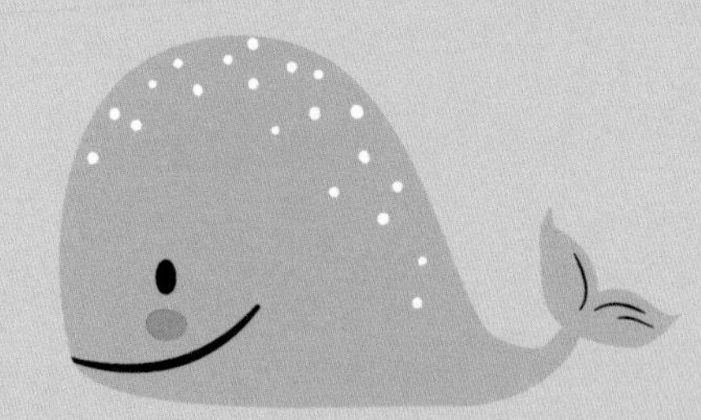

This month you learned how to . . .

We did lots of . . .

You're growing!
This is how much you grew!

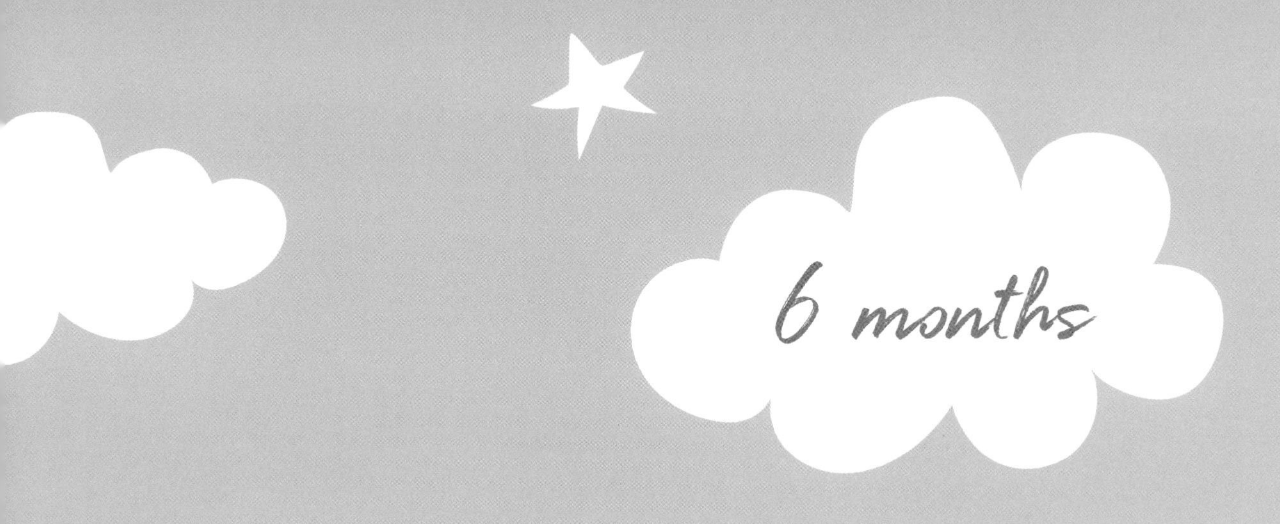
6 months

PHOTO
Memories

We did lots of . . . ________________________

____

____

____

____

____

____

____

This month you learned how to . . .

____

____

____

____

____

____

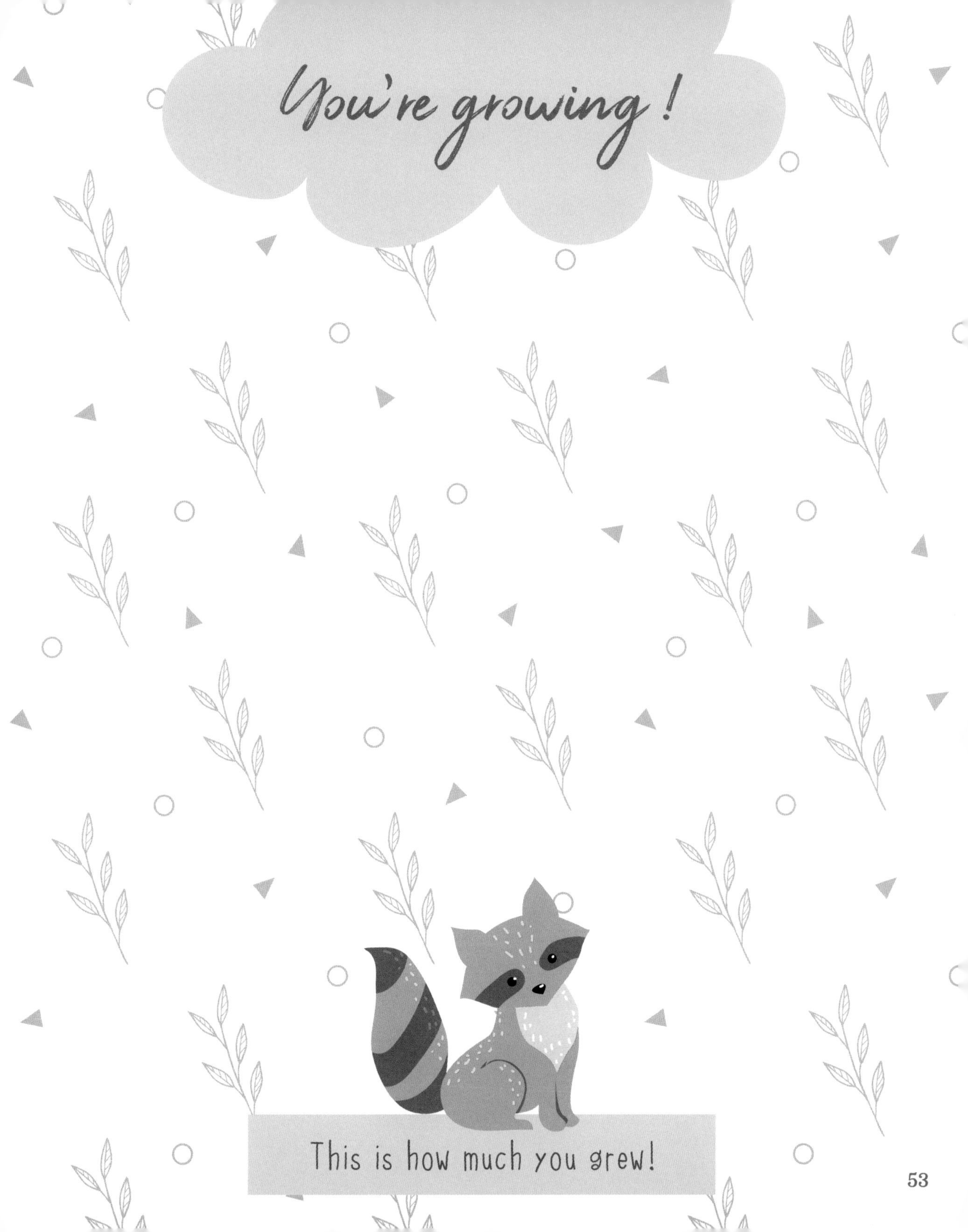
You're growing!
This is how much you grew!

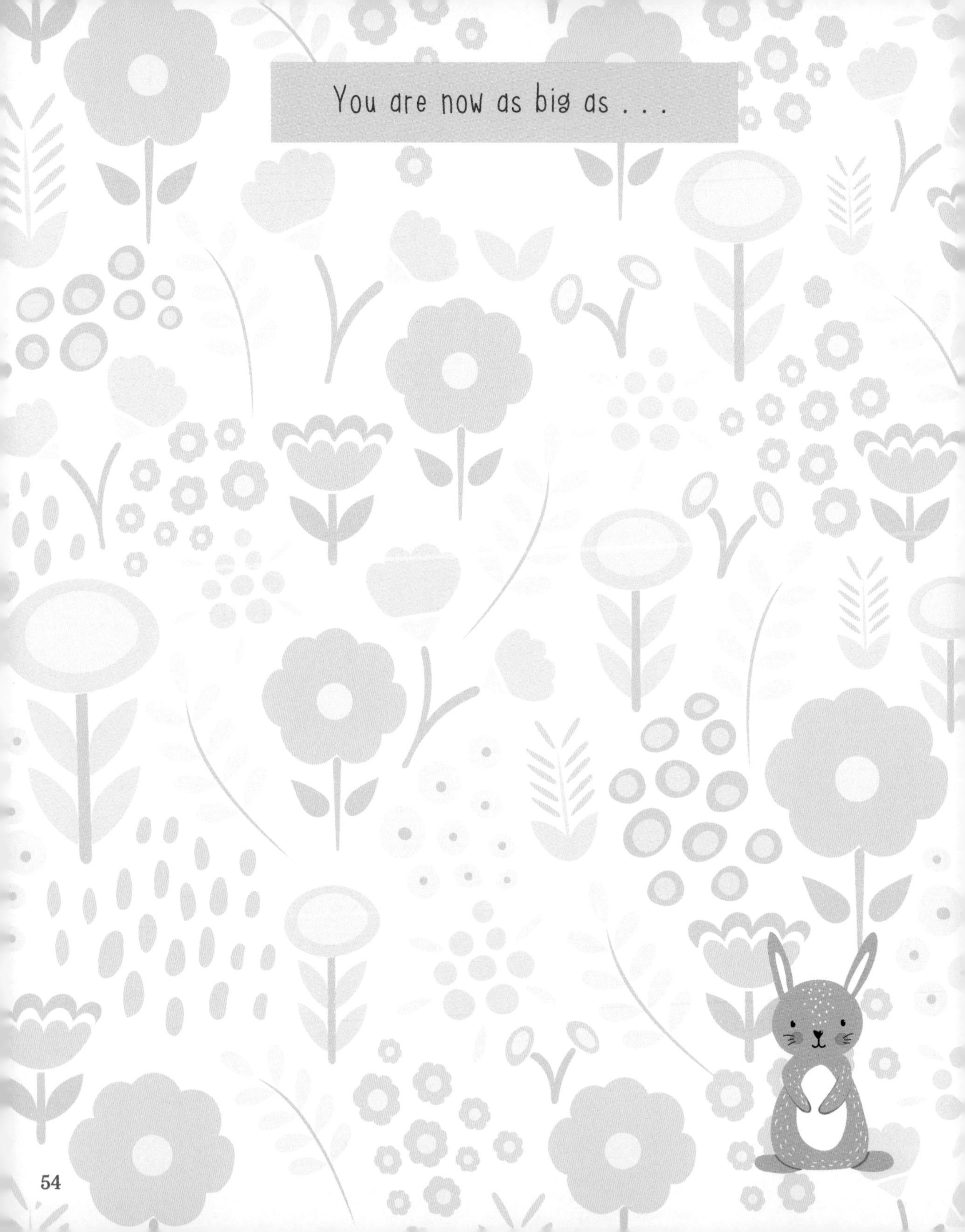

You are now as big as . . .

7 months

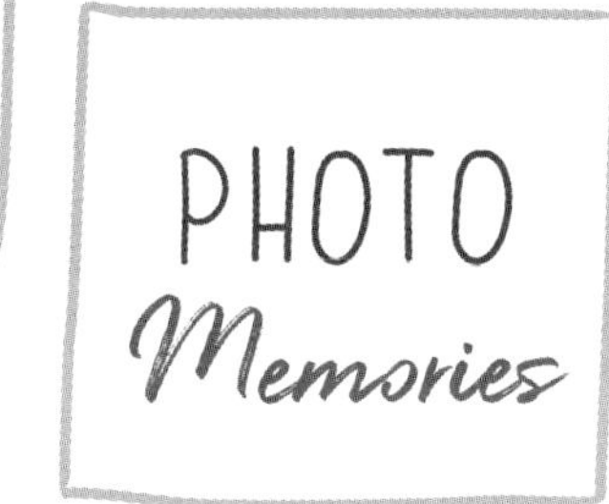

This month you learned how to . . .

We did lots of . . .

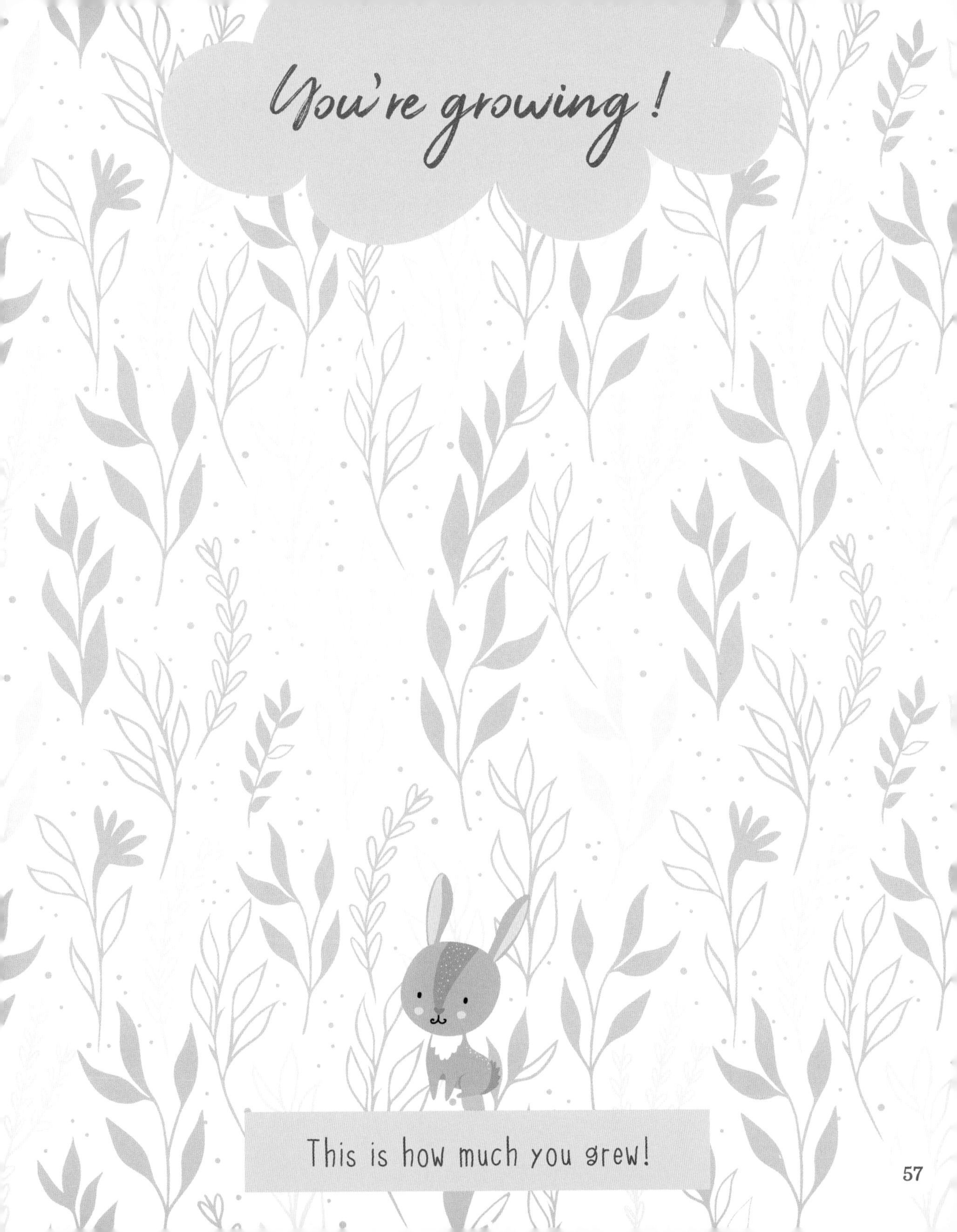
You're growing!
This is how much you grew!

8 months

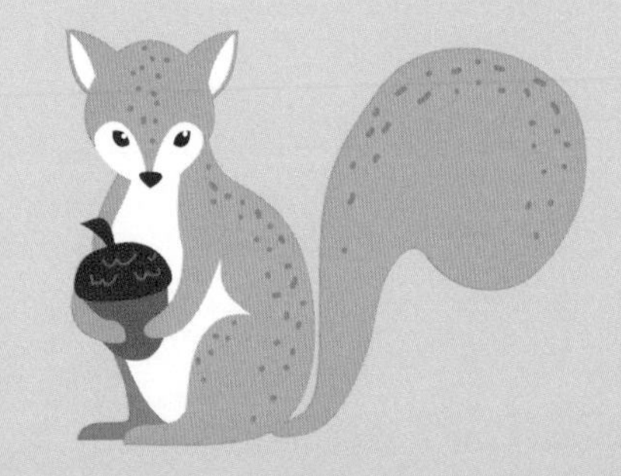

This month you learned how to . . .

We did lots of . . .

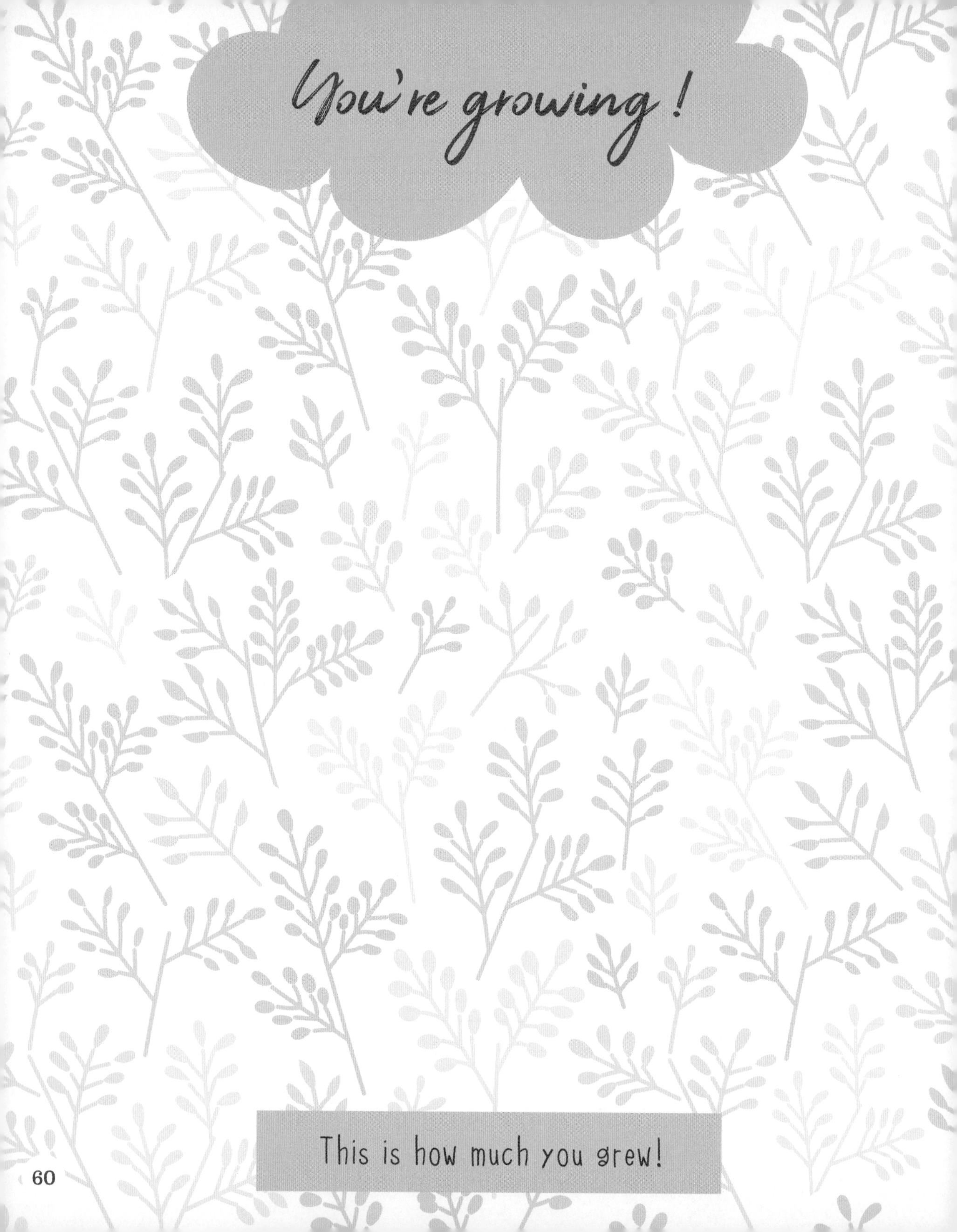
You're growing!
This is how much you grew!

9 months

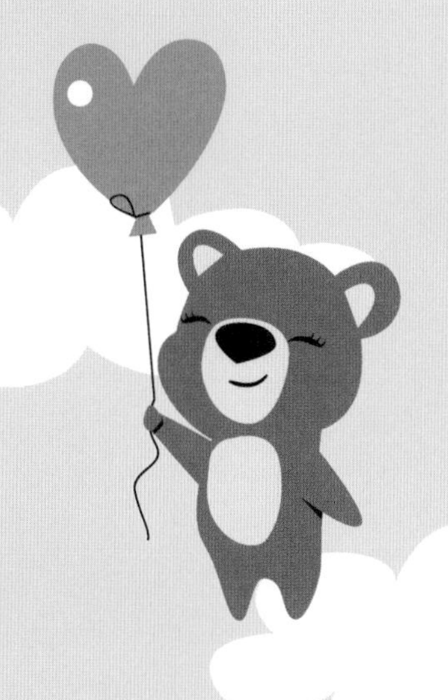

This month you learned how to . . .

We did lots of . . .

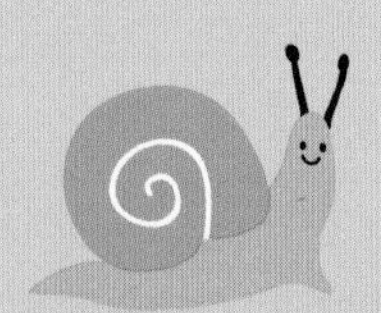

You're growing!
This is how much you grew!

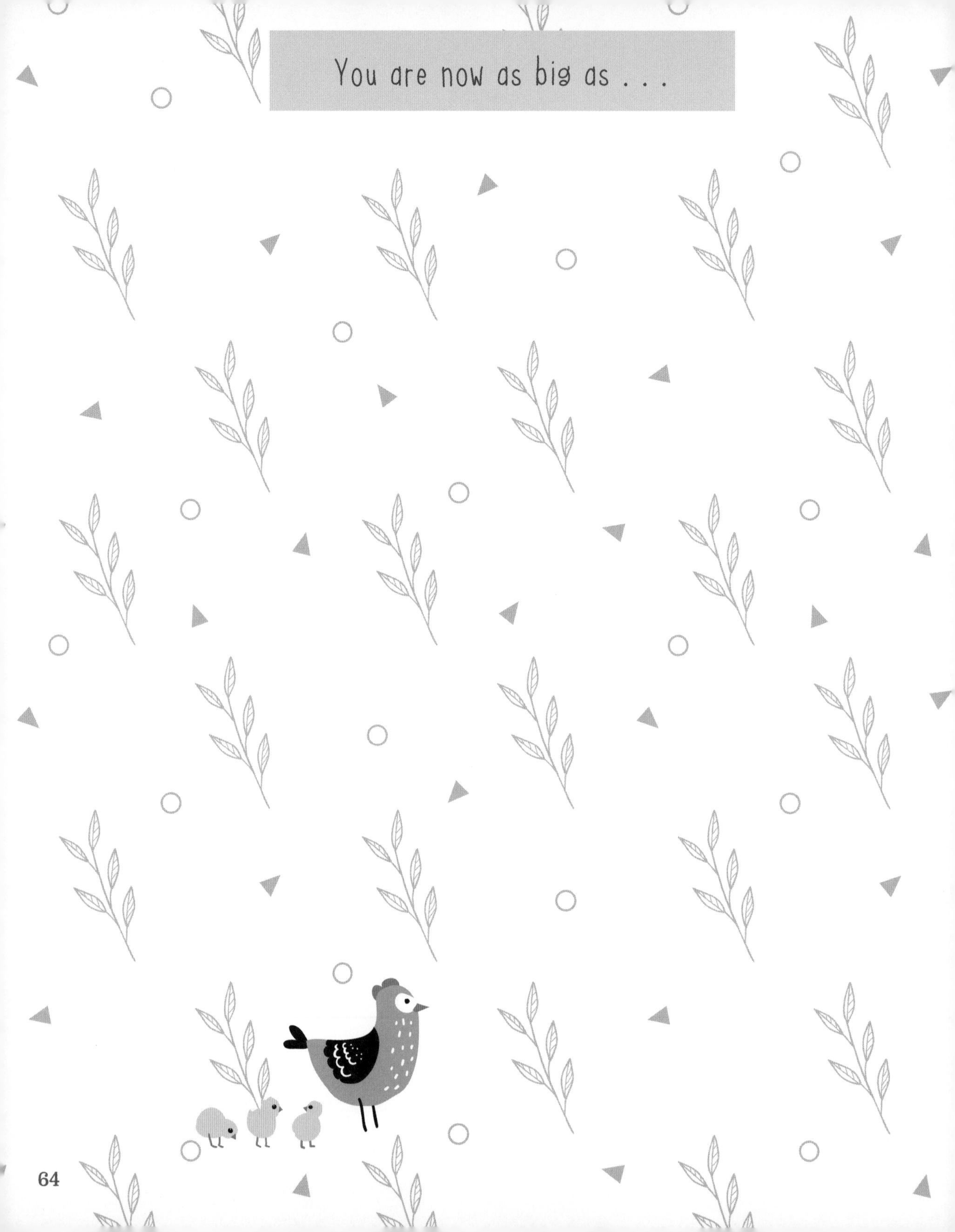

You are now as big as . . .

10 months

PHOTO
Memories

This month you learned how to . . .

We did lots of . . .

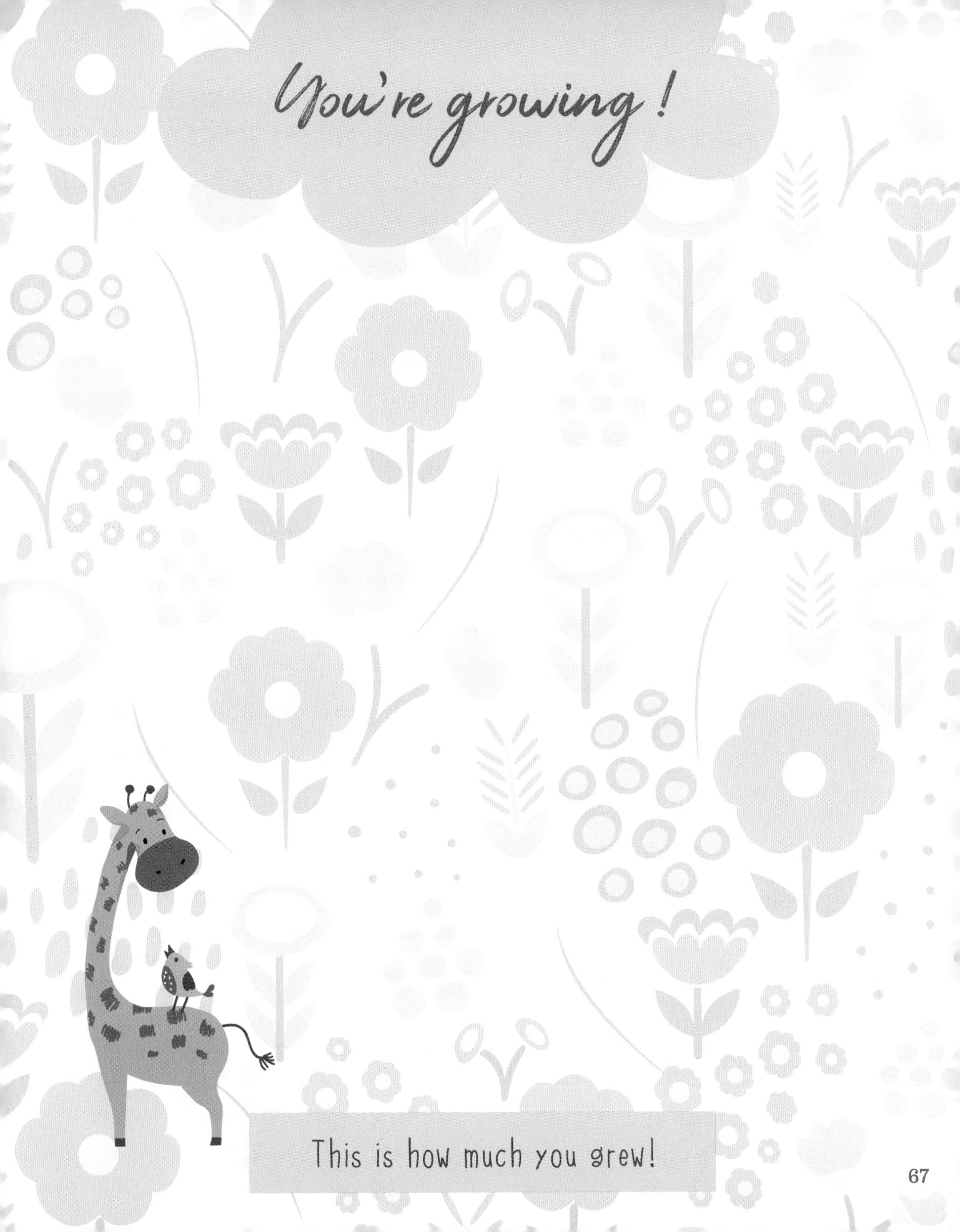
You're growing!
This is how much you grew!

11 months

This month you learned how to . . .

We did lots of . . .

You're growing!
This is how much you grew!

12 months

PHOTO
Memories

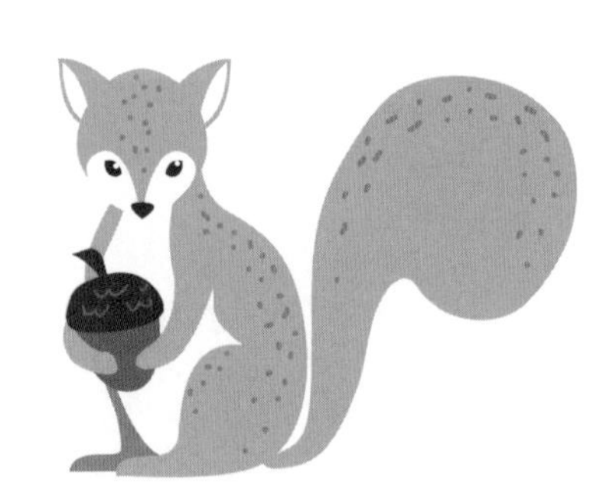

Things that make you happy . . .

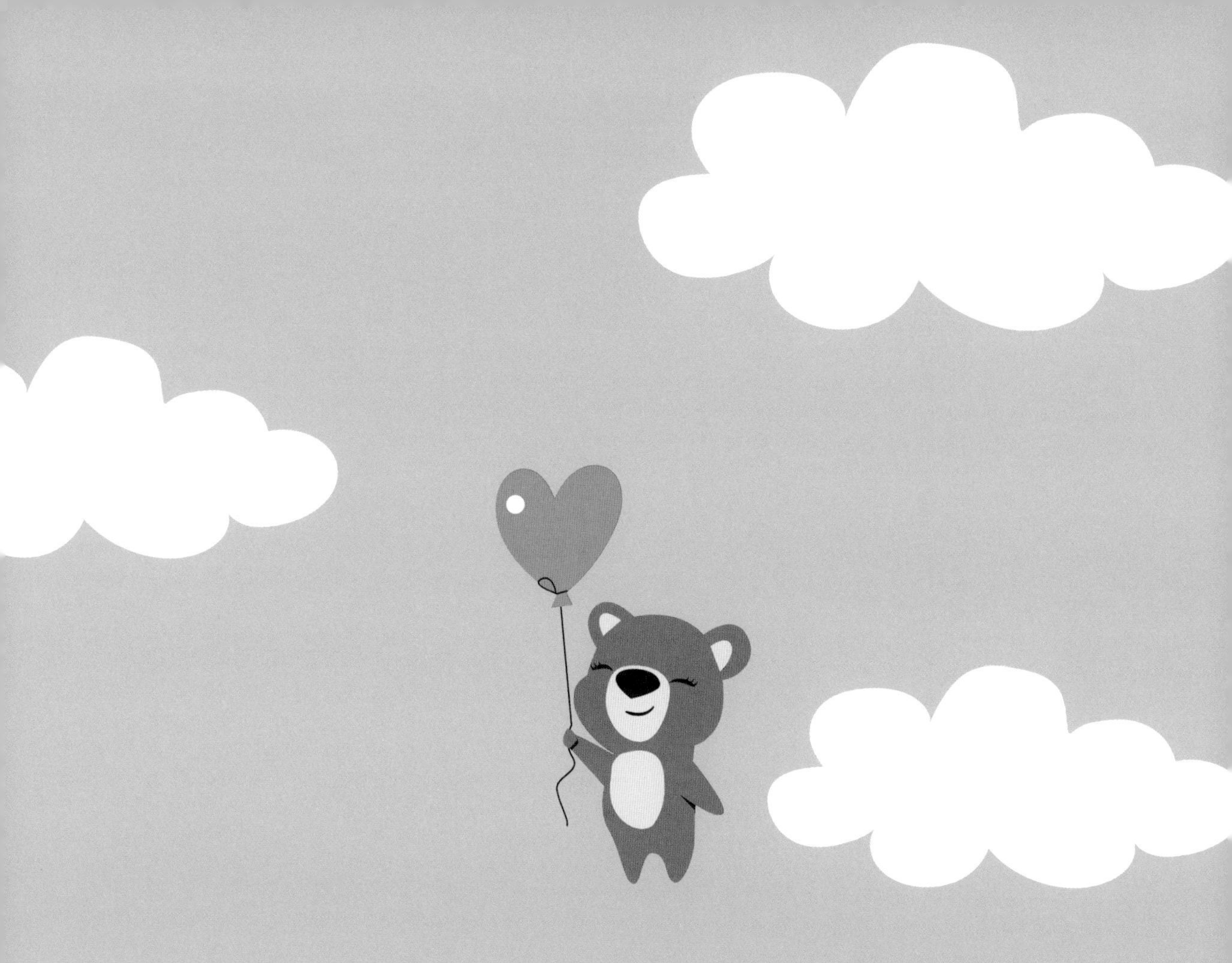

This month you learned how to . . .

We did lots of . . .

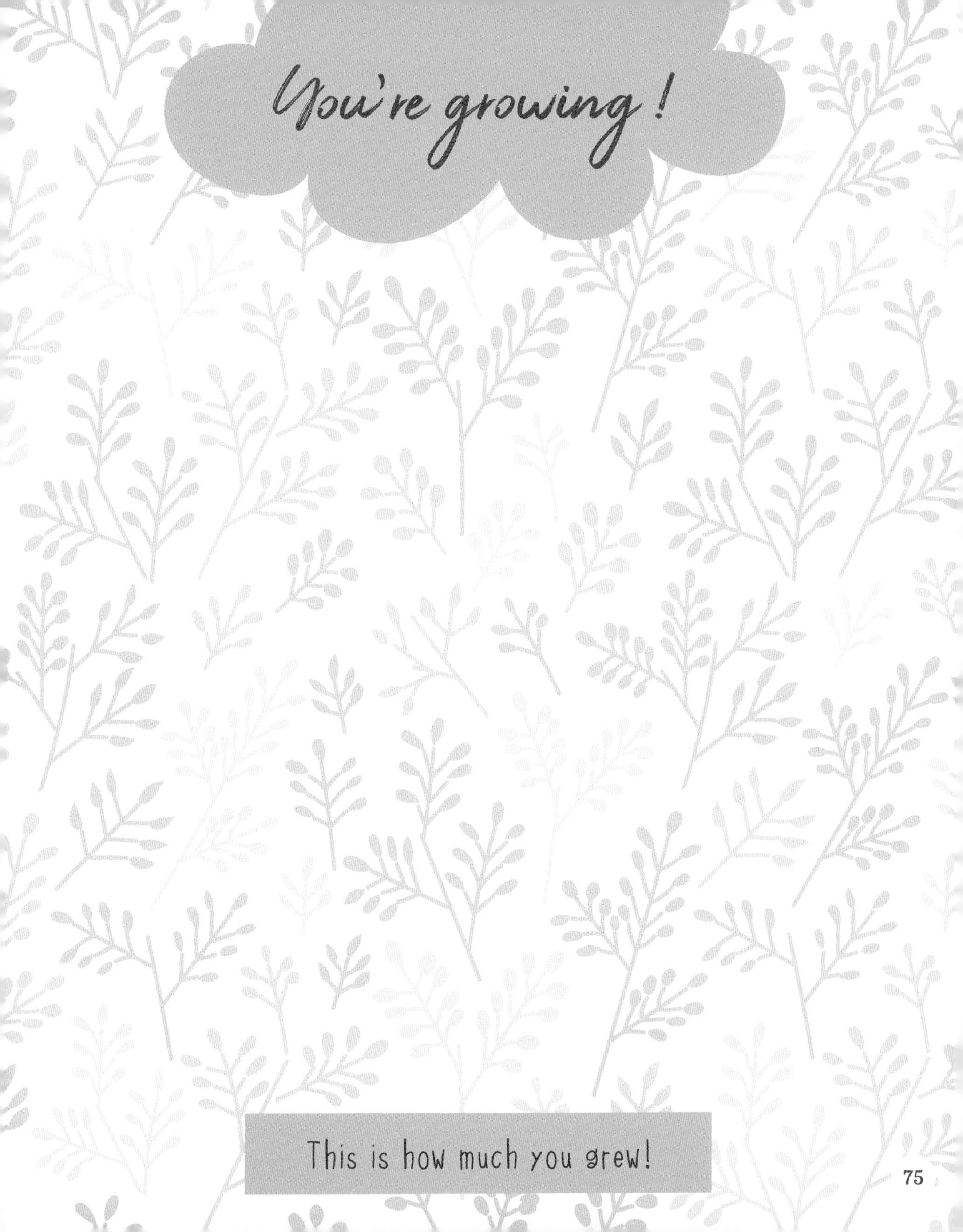
You're growing!
This is how much you grew!

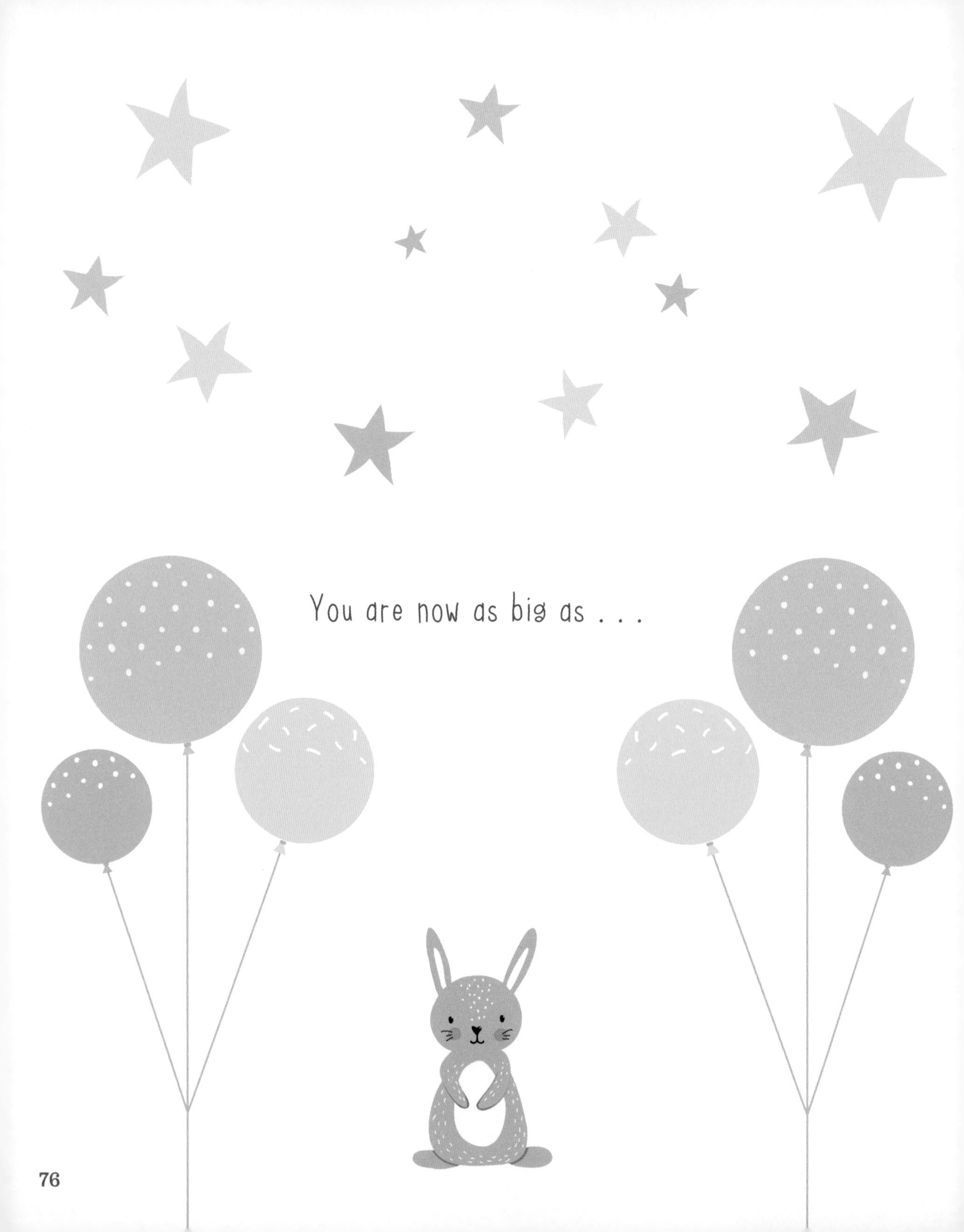
You are now as big as . . .

Your first birthday!

This was your cake!

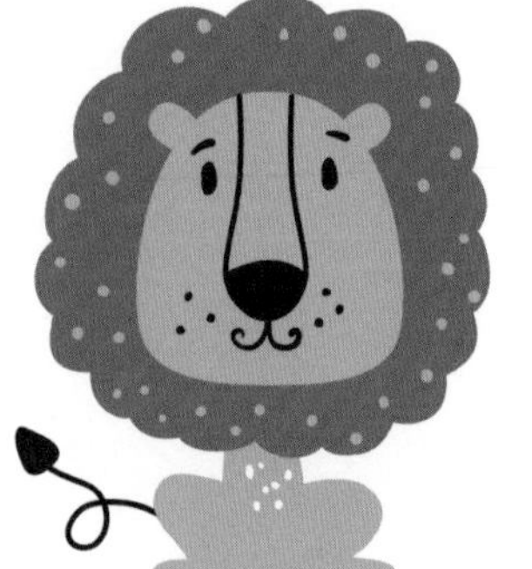

These were your presents!

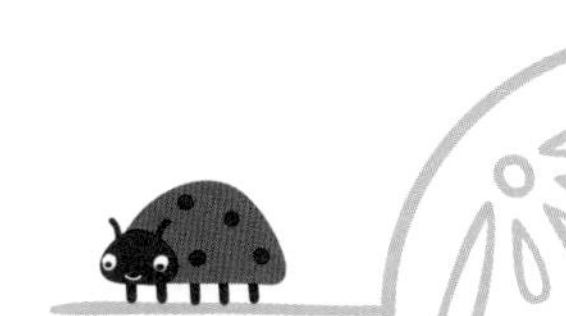

The people who came!

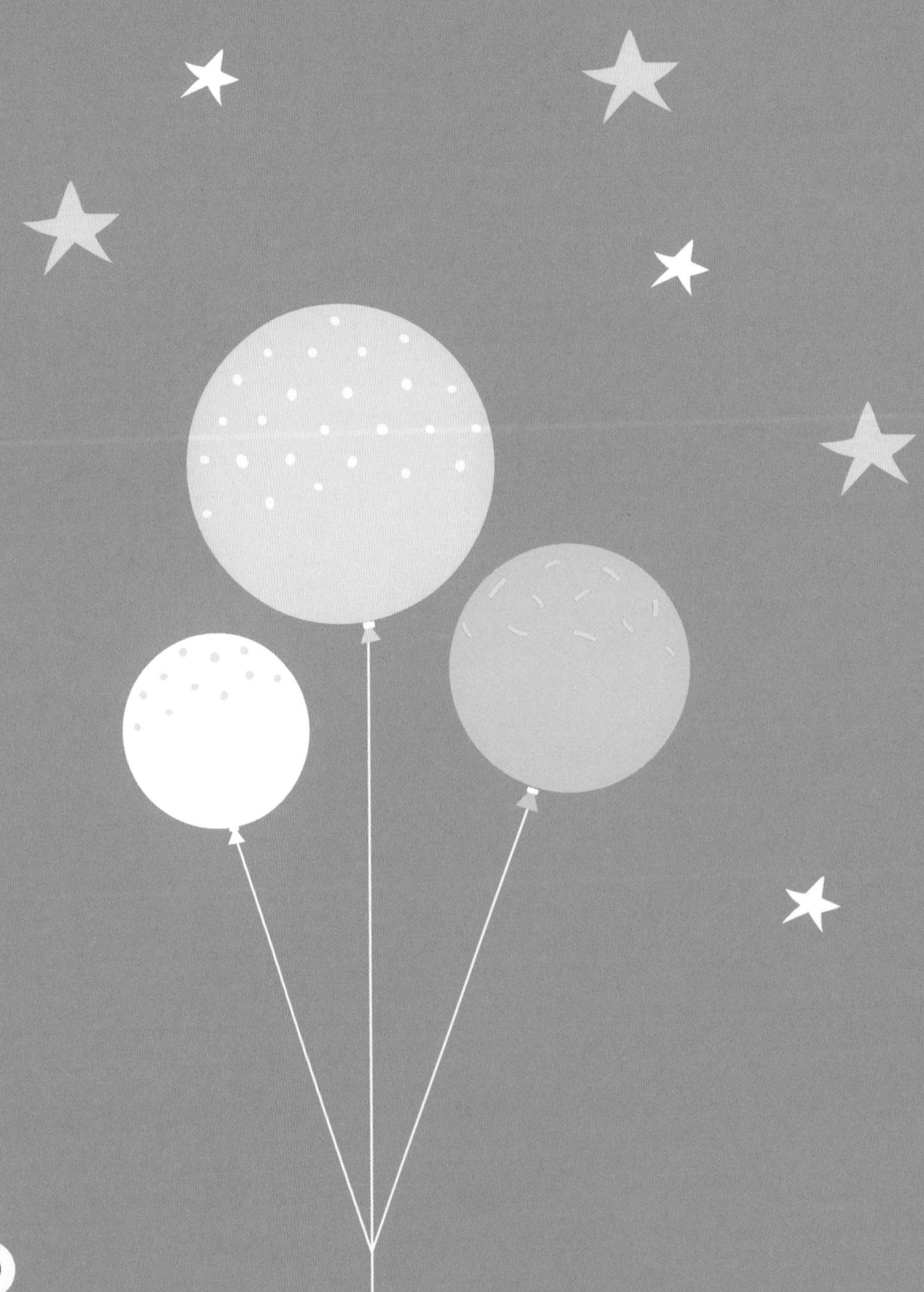

This is how you spent your day

PHOTO
Memories

Special occasions

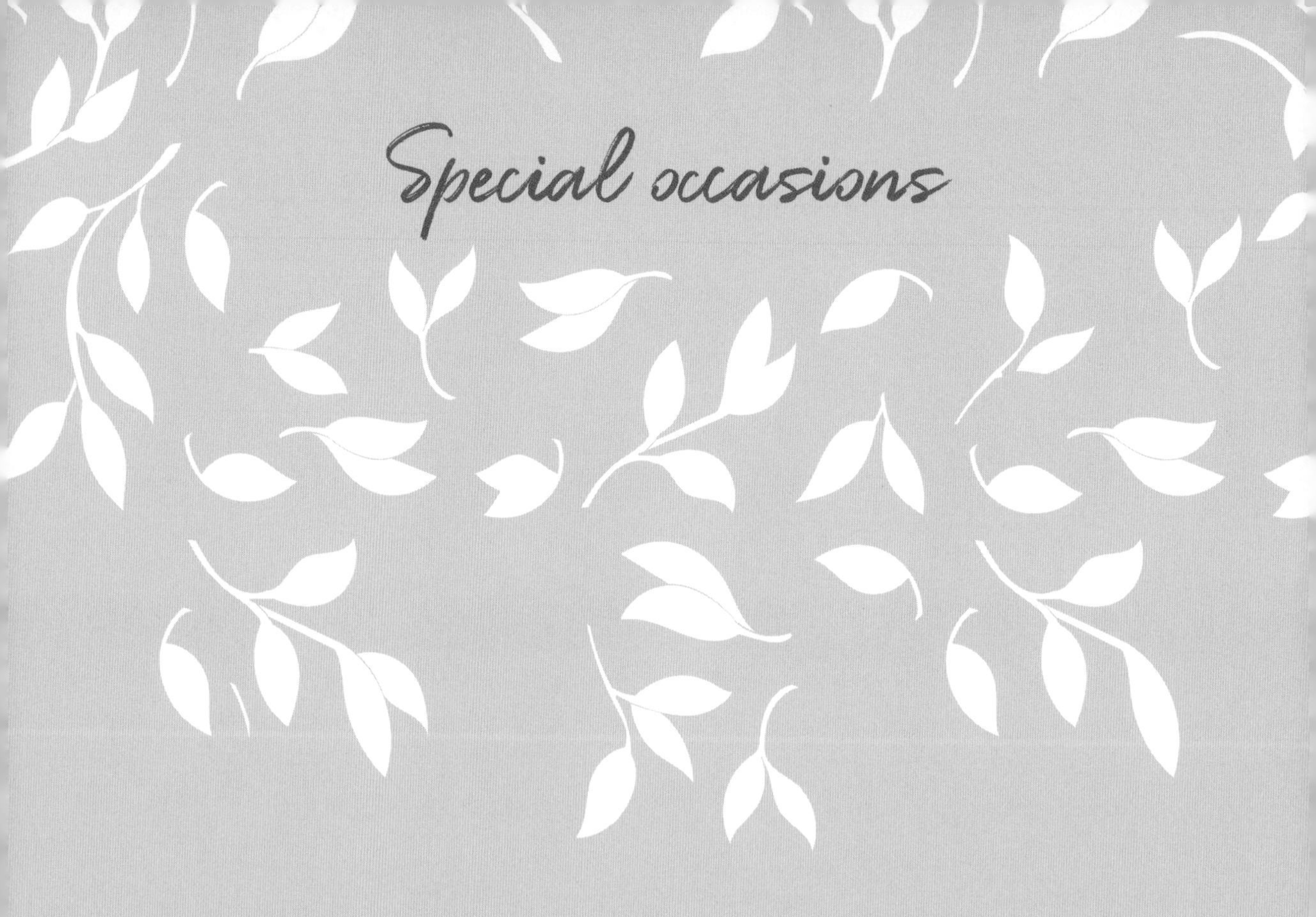

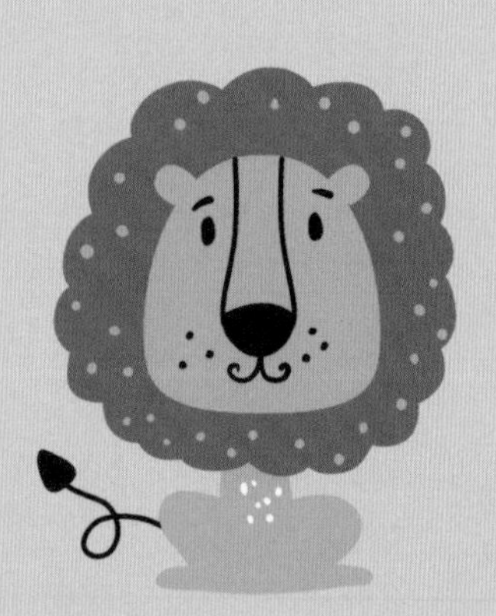

When was this?

Who was there?

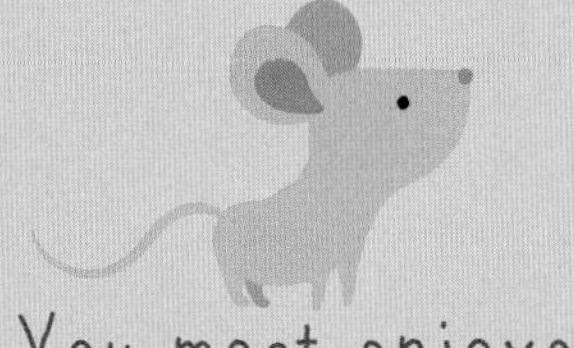

You most enjoyed . . .

Special occasions

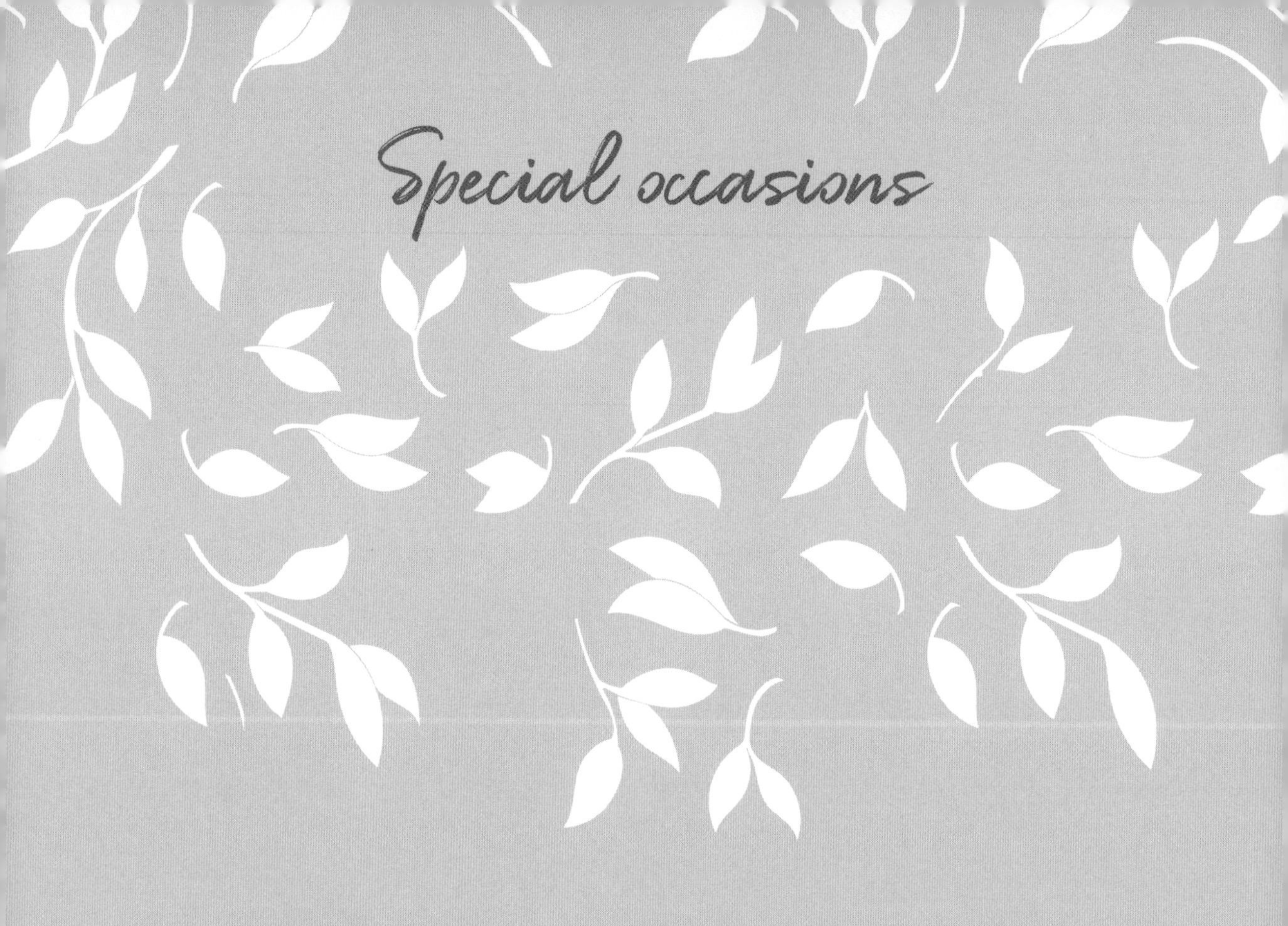

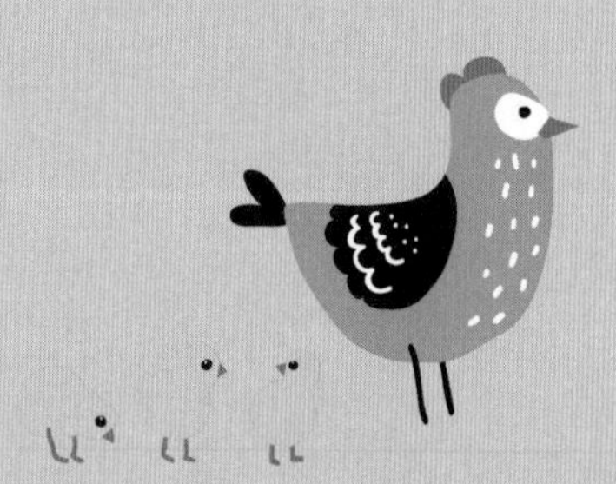

When was this?

Who was there?

You most enjoyed . . .

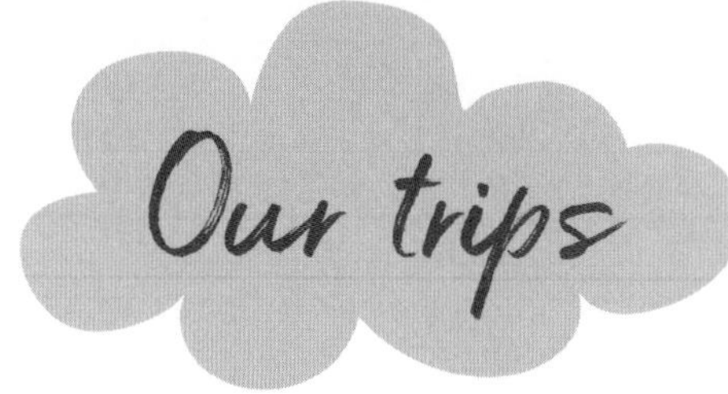

Our trips

Where?

When?

We went with . . .

The best part was . . .

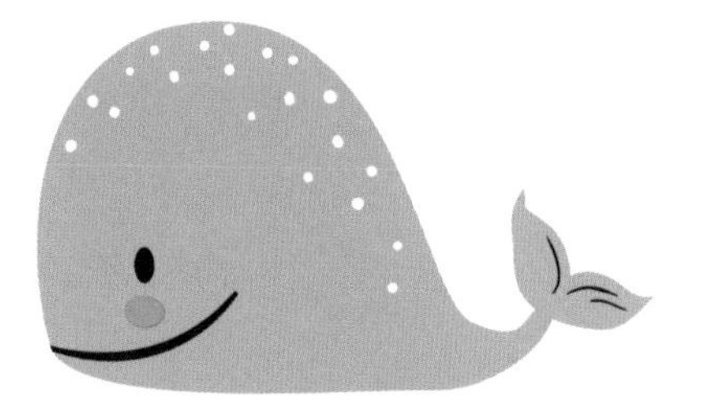

Our trips

Where?

When?

We went with . . .

The best part was . . .

Our best

PICTURES

from this year

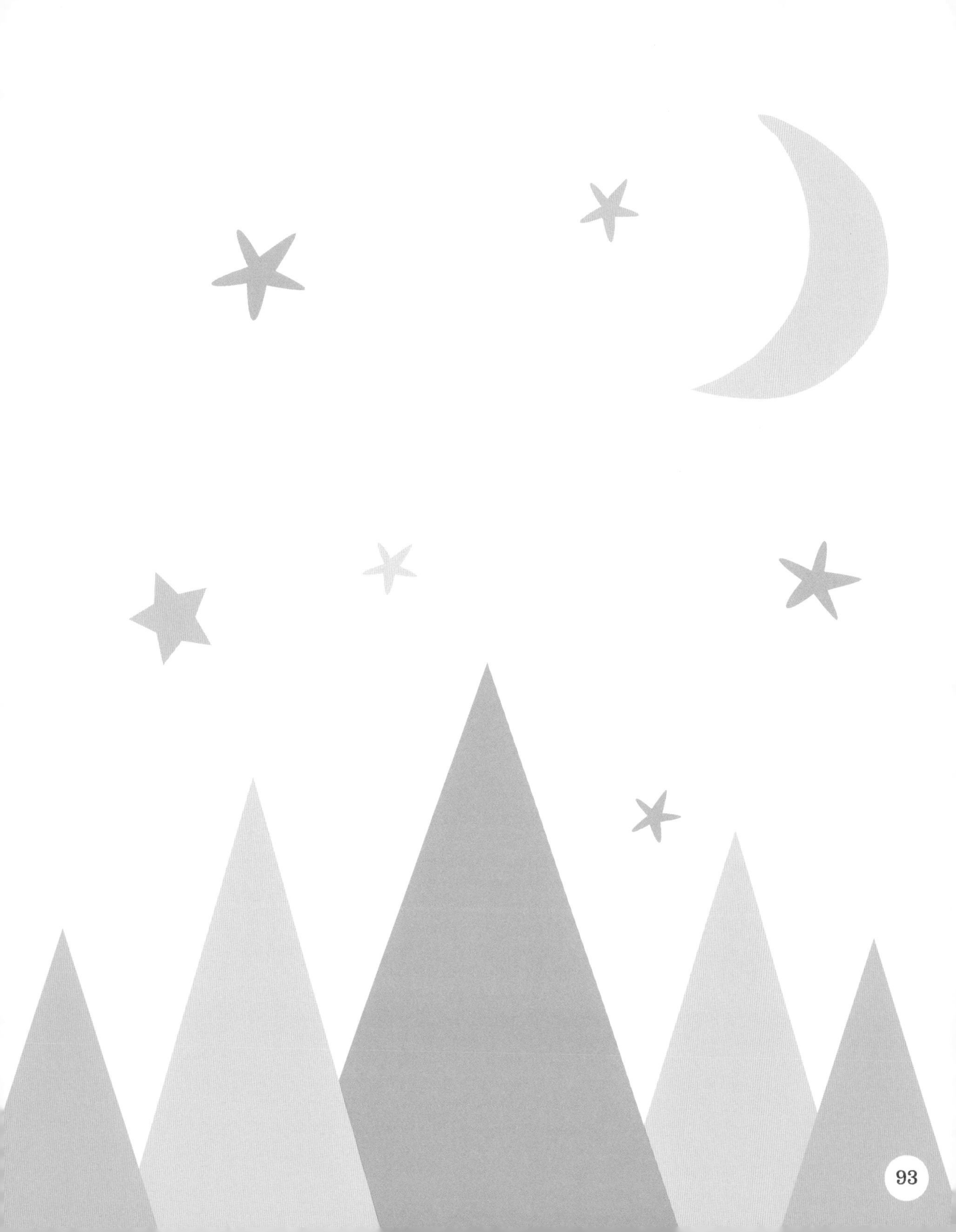

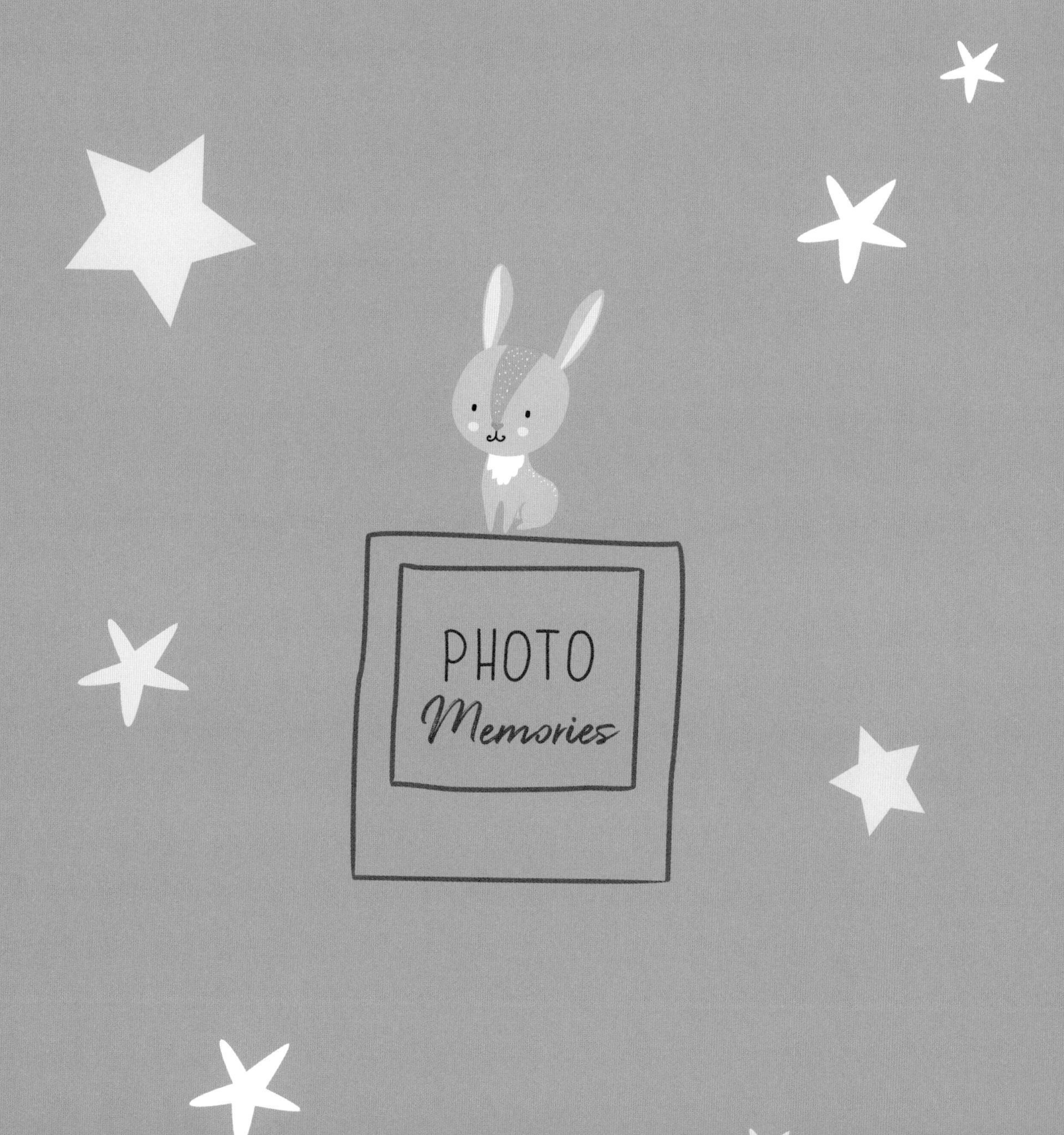
PHOTO
Memories